Taking Charge of Arthritis

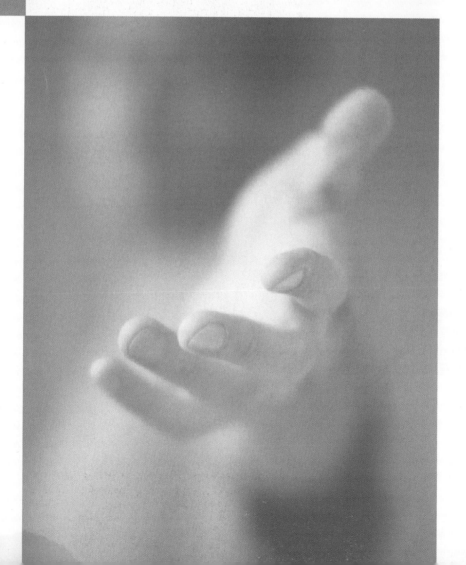

Contents

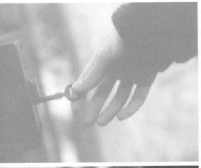
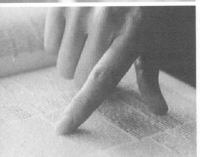
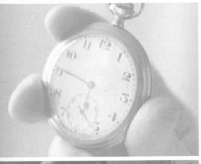
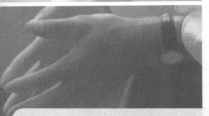

Taking Charge of
Arthritis

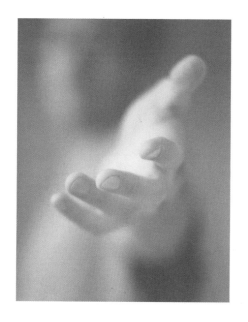

READER'S DIGEST

Published by
The Reader's Digest Association Limited
London · New York · Sydney · Montreal

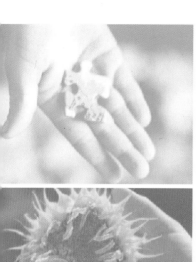

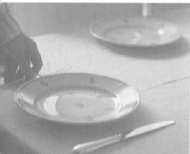

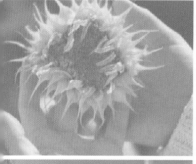

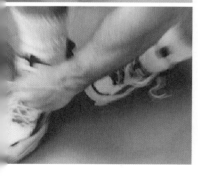

Consultant
Dr Vince Forte

Project Editor
Rachel Warren Chadd

Art Editor
Kate Harris

Assistant Editors
Jill Steed, Celia Coyne

Researcher
Caroline North

Proofreaders
Barry Gage, Rosemary Wighton

Reader's Digest, London

Editorial Director Cortina Butler
Art Director Nick Clark
Executive Editor Julian Browne
Managing Editor Alastair Holmes
Picture Resource Manager Martin Smith
Style Editor Ron Pankhurst

Book Production Manager Fiona McIntosh
Pre-press Accounts Manager Penelope Grose

Origination Colour Systems Limited, London
Printing and Binding Cayfosa Quebecor, Barcelona, Spain

Reader's Digest USA

Editorial Director Wayne Kalyn
Production Technology Manager Douglas A. Croll
Editorial Manager Christine R. Guido

Contributors

Writer Larry Katzenstein
Design Spinning Egg Design Group
Senior Designer Martha Grossman
Illustrators Articulate Graphics, Hugo Cruz, Linda Frichtell
Indexer Robert Elwood

Medical Consultants

Eddys Disla, MD
Associate chief of rheumatology, Cabrini Medical Center, New York,
and a fellow of the American College of Rheumatology

Dr. John Hassall, F.R.A.C.P.,
Emeritus consultant in rheumatology,
Royal Prince Alfred Hospital, Sydney, Australia

About this book

If you consider the hundreds of books on arthritis that have been published over the years, you might wonder if another book on the subject is really necessary. Surely those who suffer from arthritis can find out everything they need to know from the vast library already devoted to the condition?

Or maybe not. *Taking Charge of Arthritis* contains the latest, most relevant information about managing and preventing arthritis and – most importantly – provides practical advice and strategies to help you to apply that information to your benefit. This is – in a nutshell – news that you can use. If your goal is to treat, prevent or overcome the chronic pain of osteoarthritis or the related inflammatory condition, rheumatoid arthritis, this book will give you the facts, the plan and the inspiration to accomplish your aim.

Taking Charge of Arthritis is, essentially, two books in one. If you're the sort of person who likes to follow a programme, this book has come up with a very successful one for you. Based on the Arthritis Self-Help Course pioneered by Stanford University in the USA and adapted for a British audience with advice from Arthritis Care, who run the similar Arthritis Self-Management Course, our programme will give you the steps and motivation to overcome your pain and disability and to lead a richer, fuller life.

On the other hand, if you are the type of person who is averse to programmes and who prefers to pick and choose what's right for you, this book will also work like a charm. Organizations including the Arthritis Research Campaign and the British Society for Rheumatology have also helped us to ensure that the book contains accurate, up-to-the-minute information that you can use to help you to achieve a measure of freedom from your condition.

Whether it be a new arthritis drug or alternative therapy that has been in the news, or the proven benefits of losing weight and getting exercise, *Taking Charge of Arthritis* has the details.

If you have arthritis and are simply trying to cope with the condition, it is time to raise your sights. You really can control your arthritis – to a greater degree than you ever imagined.

Foreword

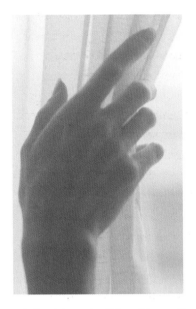

The treatment of arthritis has entered a new era. Huge progress has been made over the past decade and exciting advances in research have led to the development of therapies which are now much more effective. The doctor patient relationship is also changing and the recognized ideal is now a true partnership, which is especially important for long-term conditions such as arthritis. A good doctor will take the time to develop a relationship and will be able to discuss the best possible treatments. Patients, too, must learn as much as they can about their condition and be willing to try what is recommended and to meet challenges posed by the doctor or other members of the treatment team.

I am often struck by how differently the people I see deal with their condition. Even though individuals may be affected physically in a similar way, some continue with their work and daily life as normally as possible, refusing to let their arthritis beat them, while others cope less well, suffer more pain and become more physically limited by their condition. There is no doubt in my mind that the patients who manage better are those who have a more positive attitude towards their disease; an integral part of that is learning about their arthritis and understanding it.

Getting information is now much easier thanks to the wealth of material available on the internet. Unfortunately, all that information can be confusing, overwhelming and sometimes frightening, as it is not always explained simply or put into context and often aimed at medical professionals rather than patients. There should be no such confusion or concern with *Taking Charge of Arthritis*. This book is accurately researched and while it contains an astonishing amount of facts and other information, it is clearly written and explained and, in my view, is an excellent starting point for people with arthritis who want to manage their condition more effectively and make the most of their contact with their doctors.

The impact arthritis can have cannot be underestimated. While some severe forms may cause life-threatening illness, in most cases arthritis does not kill you but it can certainly take away your life. Activities that were once almost effortless, such as dressing, climbing stairs and even eating, can become tasks that have to be planned for and require extra time and even assistance. Knowing what to expect from arthritis helps people to deal – both mentally and physically – with potential problems, enabling them to stay active and participate in work as well as leisure pursuits, thereby controlling their disease.

One of my patients is a 23-year-old woman who was diagnosed with rheumatoid arthritis five years ago. She has one of the most severe forms of the disease I have ever come across in 15 years of practising rheumatology, and has undergone many different types of therapy. In the early days of her arthritis, she had flares severe enough to hospitalize her for days at a time.

Despite this, she remains cheerful and active, holds down a full-time job and has a long-term relationship. Recent X-rays of her hands and feet show none of the damage to the joints normally expected in this form of arthritis. She may have many years of arthritis ahead but her story so far is a success, thanks to her determination to maintain her physical fitness and mobility, and her willingness to persist and co-operate with the sometimes onerous and intensive treatment regimes necessary to control her disease.

While medical advances in the treatment of arthritis are partly responsible for controlling her disease, there is little doubt that the partnership between doctor and a well educated and motivated patient is also the key to success in overcoming arthritis.

Dr. Jeremy Camilleri, BSc FRCP
Consultant Rheumatologist and Clinical Advisor
to the Arthritis Research Campaign

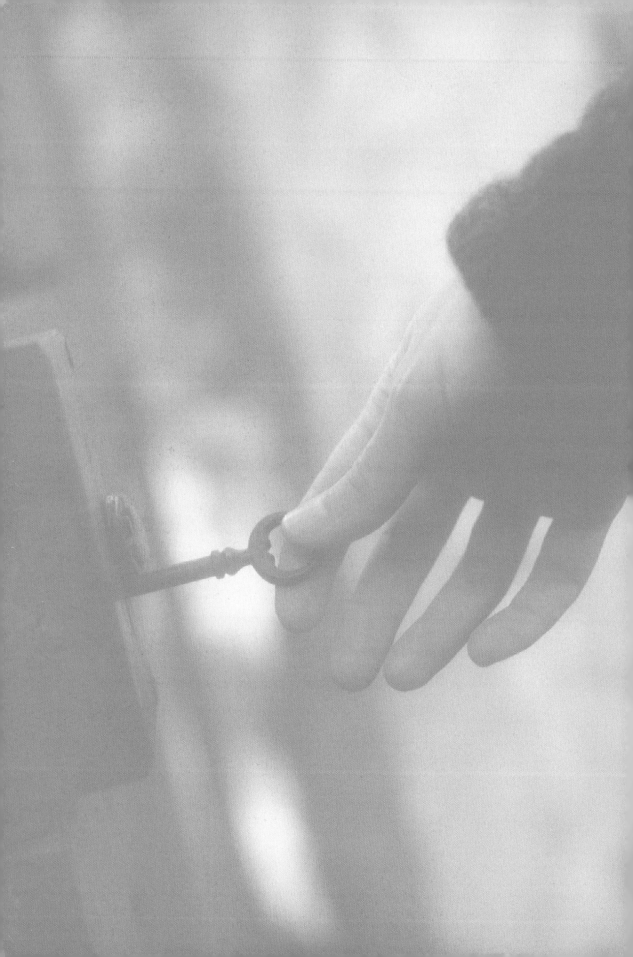

1

Confronting the problem

If you have arthritis and have been

concentrating on simply coping with

your condition, it is time to raise your

sights: you are capable of doing

much better. You can control your

arthritis to a much greater degree

than you have ever imagined.

Attitude is almost everything

Since arthritis is a chronic disease, many patients resign themselves to a 'life sentence' of painful joints and the disability they can cause. Such a defeatist attitude practically guarantees that they won't get better and may get a lot worse – because when it comes to arthritis, mind really does matter.

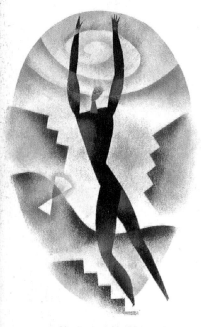

SELF-EMPOWERMENT The belief in your ability to organize and devise a course of action that will result in mastering a situation. In short, controlling your own destiny.

The confidence to overcome Thousands of people who suffer from arthritis have discovered a simple yet powerful truth that can provide hope and strength to just about anyone who develops the condition: the most successful patients, the ones who go on to live richer, fuller lives, are the ones who are most confident they can overcome the limitations of their disease. Researchers have studied many patients enrolled in arthritis self-help programmes to find out what behavioural changes are most important. Much to their surprise, the researchers found that successfully overcoming symptoms depended mainly on patients' confidence that they could do it.

What's more, a positive attitude was even more important to a patient's success than following a doctor's advice on treatment, nutrition or exercise. This way of thinking – the conviction that you control your destiny – is called self-empowerment.

Knowledge is power

In *Taking Charge of Arthritis*, you'll learn everything you need to know about your condition – from the newest information and insights into the causes of the condition to the latest break-throughs in conventional and alternative treatments.

But even more important, you'll learn to become an effective practitioner of self-empowerment. You'll do that by formulating an effective arthritis action strategy that incorporates the eight steps shown overleaf for taking control of your condition. They will guide you in tailoring a plan that will suit you and your particular circumstances.

Living with rheumatoid arthritis

Linda Logan is a former guesthouse manager from Renfrewshire, Scotland. She learned how to take charge of her arthritis by enrolling on Arthritis Care's self-management programme, 'Challenging Arthritis' and found the course so helpful that she now teaches it to others. She says this about her take-charge approach to her condition:

'I signed up for the course about seven years after I was diagnosed with rheumatoid arthritis (RA). It wasn't an easy decision because I'm not one for groups, normally. I have a great relationship with my GP and she recommended the Arthritis Care course to me. I deliberated about it and put it off for almost two years.'

When her condition was first diagnosed, Linda felt desperate, thinking life wasn't worth living, but she gradually learned to cope with her RA and was doing well at the time her GP suggested the course. She had found the right drugs to help her and that suited her well, and had even had a course of hydrotherapy, so why change? Linda says: 'It sounds strange, but at the time I thought no one could tell me anything I didn't already know.'

However, curiosity got the better of her and Linda decided to give it a go. 'I was so surprised,' she says. 'I really quite liked it! There was a real mix of people there and I actually felt comfortable, so much so that I felt able to say things I had never told anyone before.

'Having arthritis is very hard because you know it is forever and you really put yourself through the mill thinking about that. The course shows you that a positive attitude about arthritis can really help you to take charge of it. It teaches you how to adapt your life successfully and how to pace yourself.

"... a positive attitude can really help you ..."

'One of the most important things I learned on the course was how to get enjoyment out of life again. Life is too short, not to enjoy it, and it's all too easy to forget that when you have a chronic illness. The course really helped me to put the fun back into my life. I found that just talking to others and sharing similar experiences spurred me on. I now know that my life really is worth living.'

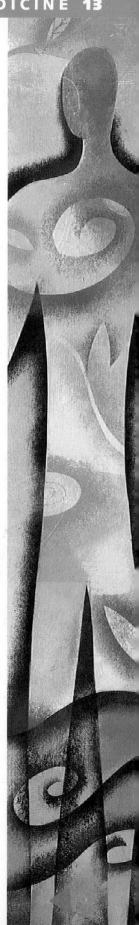

If your goal is to climb the stairs unaided, you *can* make it to the top, slowly but surely. Or if you have trouble rising from a chair after sitting down, you *can* achieve a painless liftoff. It's a matter of assessing your problem, setting reasonable goals, and then working to achieve those goals. You will be able to measure your progress in the form of reduced pain, greater mobility, and enhanced well-being.

> ◗ **FACT** Arthritis is often thought of as a problem of old age. But nearly three out of every five patients are under 65.

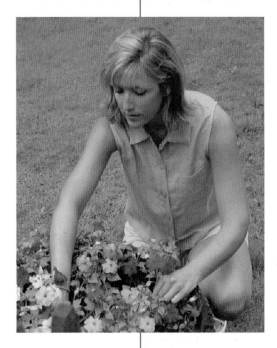

The eight steps for overcoming arthritis

This self-help approach has already liberated thousands of arthritis patients from a life of pain and disability. How? Because at the core of the plan is an incontrovertible premise: no one cares about your welfare as much as you do. Not your doctor, your family or your friends.

As many patients have found out, thoroughly educating yourself about your condition and the treatments that are available to you is a giant step toward that liberation. Just because you have a chronic disease doesn't mean that it has to rule your life. There are ways to alleviate and lessen the effects of your condition, and most of them are commonsense and quite obvious, once they're pointed out.

Digesting the information in *Taking Charge of Arthritis* and then incorporating these eight important steps into your daily life will give you the power and ability to gain the upper hand over your arthritis.

1 Get to know your problem

The more you know about a problem, the better you will be able to deal with it. And the better acquainted you are with arthritis, the better equipped you will be to overcome it. This isn't a very profound insight, but it is a very powerful one. In *Taking Charge of Arthritis*, you'll learn the answers to vitally important questions about your particular type of arthritis, such as 'What causes it?' 'How is it diagnosed?' 'What are the best treatments available?'

This book is full of valuable insights that will help you to analyse your individual problem. Is pain the most troublesome symptom you experience? If so, how bad is it? Is it worse in the morning or later in the day? By answering these and other questions, you'll be able to develop an effective anti-arthritis programme tailored to your needs.

2 Choose your long-term goal

Chances are you want to resume a much-loved activity – going for a walk on the beach or playing with the children or grand-children, for example – that arthritis has taken away from you. The best goals are specific, well-defined ones such as 'I want to be able to walk a mile without knee pain.' It's easier to motivate yourself to achieve a specific goal than a vague goal and it's also easier to tell whether you have attained it. Whatever it is, carving out a clear-cut goal can provide the motivation you need to jump-start your arthritis self-management plan.

3 Decide on a strategy

Once you have your goal, you need a treatment strategy to help you to reach it. Certainly, there is no shortage of treatment approaches available. Books, websites, news segments on the latest arthritis treatments – there is a confusing glut of information to contend with. Do you want to eliminate the pain in your arthritic knee? If so, you could take a number of approaches including weight loss, an exercise programme, or using anti-inflammatory drugs. Do you want to take the load off your knees by losing 20lb? You could skip high-calorie desserts and cheeses, begin an exercise programme, decrease the size of your portions at meal times or take a calorie-controlled lunch to work instead of eating out. Or you could combine several of these approaches into your overall strategy.

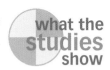

what the studies show

Arthritis patients who actively participate in their own care, report less pain, require fewer doctor visits and enjoy a better quality of life. In one recent study of participants in an arthritis self-help programme, patients who completed the programme reported nearly a 20 per cent reduction in pain and 40 per cent fewer doctor visits than non-participants. And the benefits of participating in the programme lasted for four years.

The many faces of arthritis

Arthritis is not a single disease but actually encompasses a total of 127 separate disorders. They include those you're probably familiar with such as osteoarthritis, rheumatoid arthritis and gout, as well as much rarer types such as psoriatic arthritis (see Chapter 2). Although many of these 100-plus disorders have very different causes and symptoms, they do share a common feature: all of them involve inflammation of the joints. Indeed, the term 'arthritis' comes from the Greek words *arthron* (which means joint) and *itis* (which means inflammation).

No goal worth achieving can be reached overnight or without effort. An effective anti-arthritis strategy will require some work or even some sacrifices (forgoing those tempting desserts, for example), but reaching your goal will ultimately make it all worthwhile.

4 Draw up your weekly take-charge plan

For someone with arthritis, that old Chinese saying, 'A journey of a thousand miles must begin with a single step,' is literally and figuratively true. In creating your weekly take-charge plan you need to decide on a short-term goal and then assign yourself specific actions for achieving that goal.

> A positive attitude may be even more important to a patient's success than following a doctor's advice on treatment, nutrition or exercise.

If, for example, you decide that you want to lose 20lb, your take-charge plan might call for a short-term goal of losing a pound a week. Then you get down to specific weight-loss actions – eliminating fattening desserts, for example, or walking to burn up calories. If you manage to complete those actions with relatively little effort, you can consider writing in slightly more ambitious actions for next week's plan.

Build a team It's wise to be inclusive when drawing up your take-charge plan. Ask for your doctor's advice, especially if you haven't yet been diagnosed with arthritis or don't know what kind you have. Many people assume that their aches and pains stem from arthritis, but sometimes their problems are being caused by something else entirely, such as an adverse reaction to a drug, an infection or even a malignancy. So if you're not sure whether you have arthritis, now is the time to see your doctor – before trying to manage a condition you might not even have!

If you have been diagnosed with arthritis, work closely with your doctor to draw up a management plan that will suit your circumstances and put it into action. Try to see your doctor and you as a team: a good partnership with your doctor can greatly assist you in achieving your goals.

In Chapter 4, 'Working with Your Doctor', we will tell you how to get the most out of this relationship, with advice on choosing a doctor if you need one, preparing for surgery visits, asking the right questions once you're there, and building a strong team of supporters – from your family to a physiotherapist to, possibly, an acupuncturist as well.

5 Put your take-charge plan into action

Now comes the hard part: following through on the strategy you've devised. If your goal of losing a pound over the next week calls for cutting out 500 calories per day, you may have to deny yourself that morning pastry and afternoon cappuccino.

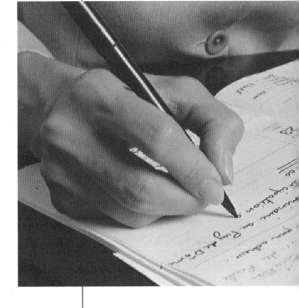

6 Monitor your progress

As the week passes, note how well you've done in completing the actions you've assigned yourself in your take-charge plan. Congratulate yourself if you've been able to stick to your plan, but try not to berate yourself if you did some backsliding. Nobody ever said that changing a habit was easy.

7 Adjust your action plan

If you don't attain the short-term goal called for in your weekly take-charge plan, work out what went wrong and identify a way to correct it. If you lost only half a pound, maybe losing a pound a week was too ambitious. Or it may have turned out that losing a pound was easy and you could safely lose a little more. Either way, you will probably need to fine-tune your action plan.

8 Build on your success

Success, as we know, is one of the best of all motivators. If you've achieved your short-term goal for one week, the momentum from that success will carry over into the following week – and inspire you to set a more ambitious goal. As you target and attain new goals, you'll find yourself actually overcoming your arthritis in the process.

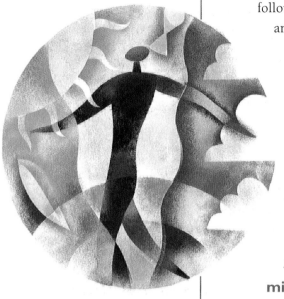

The secrets of self-treatment

As you start drawing up your self-management plan, you'll probably incorporate a variety of therapies. As you do so, it is important to bear in mind that people can vary widely in their responses to therapies.

Because no two bodies are identical, individuals with similar symptoms will respond differently to the same treatment. What helps your arthritis pain might not help someone else. Therefore be patient and open-minded as you try to assess therapies for your condition.

now and then

As recently as 20 years ago, doctors advised arthritis patients against exercising for fear that it would worsen joint damage and inflammation. But it's now recognized that moderate physical activity can be one of the most effective of all arthritis treatments.

FACT Surgery to repair or replace arthritic joints is a last resort – but can produce dramatic results. For example, surgical procedures for implanting artificial hips and knees have greatly improved in recent years and can virtually eliminate pain and disability caused by arthritis.

Help yourself As you'll learn in this book, some of the most effective anti-arthritis therapies don't involve drugs but are, instead, things you can do for yourself every day. Unfortunately, many doctors fail to recommend non-drug therapies for their arthritis patients – despite considerable evidence that such therapies can be quite effective in relieving pain and disability.

caution

Vitamin E formulations containing gamma tocopherol may actually make arthritis worse. Researchers at the University of North Carolina, USA measured blood levels of two forms of vitamin E (gamma tocopherol and alpha tocopherol) in 400 volunteers. X-rays revealed that the volunteers with high blood levels of gamma tocopherol were much more likely to have developed osteoarthritis. So avoid brands of vitamin E labelled as 'E-complex' or 'mixed tocopherols,' as they are most likely to contain gamma tocopherol. Instead look for brands with only alpha tocopherol.

Taking Charge of Arthritis gives you a practical plan for using nutrition, exercise, dietary supplements and other do-it-yourself therapies to treat your arthritis. For example, in these pages you'll find invaluable strategies and techniques to:

Lose weight

Losing just a few pounds can relieve your knee pain just as effectively as the most potent painkiller. If your goal is to lose weight, you'll learn about tried-and-trusted weight-loss strategies that will help you to lose the pounds and keep them off.

Take the right vitamins

The Framingham Osteoarthritis Study (part of the long-running Framingham Heart Study in the USA) has found that diets rich in certain vitamins may slow down the progression of osteoarthritis or even prevent the disease from occurring. *Taking Charge of Arthritis* gives you the inside information on the vitamins that can make a big difference in your condition, along with how much of each you should take.

Exercise pain away

Studies during the past decade have shown that strengthening the muscles that surround and support the joints can yield valuable results in the form of reduced pain and greater mobility. For example, strengthening your thigh muscles can dramatically relieve pain and stiffness in osteoarthritis of the knees. You'll learn about these simple exercises as well as many others, including such exotic but effective therapies as yoga and t'ai chi.

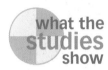

what the studies show

In a new and surprising study, people with rheumatoid arthritis who simply wrote about stressful events in their lives experienced significant reductions in their symptoms.

Learn to relax

Stress doesn't cause arthritis, but there is ample evidence that stress can worsen the condition – especially by increasing the muscle tension that can aggravate joint pain. *Taking Charge of Arthritis* suggests the best techniques for defusing the stress in your life, including the mind-body approaches that can do so much to help arthritis patients.

Take an alternative approach

Three dietary supplements have shown genuine value in treating arthritis, while other well publicized treatments waste your money and could jeopardize your health. *Taking Charge of Arthritis* takes a hard look at the science behind alternative therapies and draws conclusions about which can help you and which can harm you.

Saying 'yes' to drugs

Self-help measures may be all you need to control and overcome your arthritis, and you won't need to rely on the arsenal of arthritis drugs.

But for many people, prescription and over-the-counter drugs remain crucially important for treating their condition. In the past few years, researchers have made great strides in developing safer and better medications to battle the pain of arthritis, some of which you may not have heard about. Here's a sampling of the cutting-edge treatments you'll learn about in this book:

- **Severe rheumatoid arthritis** no longer needs to be a crippling disorder. A new class of drugs, called the disease-modifying anti-rheumatic drugs (DMARDs), has drastically changed the treatment of this highly painful, disfiguring condition. Recent studies show that these drugs may slow or even halt the joint damage that occurs in rheumatoid arthritis. The availability of these drugs should mean that many fewer patients will be crippled by their disease.

- **Three recently approved** non-steroidal anti-inflammatory drugs (NSAIDs) – Celebrex, Mobic, and Vioxx – can relieve arthritis pain and inflammation as effectively as traditional

did you know

- Smoking cigarettes can worsen the symptoms of rheumatoid arthritis and is considered to be a risk factor in triggering the disease. Smoking may cause abnormalities in the immune system of rheumatoid arthritis patients.

NSAIDs while posing much less risk of potentially fatal side effects such as stomach bleeding. And although some standard NSAIDs may damage cartilage when used regularly – something even many doctors don't know about – these three new drugs probably don't pose that risk.

● **Two revolutionary liquids** – Synvisc and Hyalan – can be injected directly into the knee joint, weekly for three to five weeks, to lubricate and nourish cartilage. Both of these recently approved substances are derived from the combs of cockerels and contain hyaluronic acid, a normal component of the joint's synovial fluid. According to recent studies, these products can relieve pain for months and may be ideal for people with osteoarthritis of the knee who've failed to respond to or couldn't tolerate other forms of treatment.

In addition, *Taking Charge of Arthritis* will also tell you about a wide range of promising treatments – from antibiotic therapy to gene therapy – now being investigated that may be available to you soon.

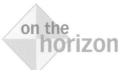

on the horizon

In 1990, a study in the *New England Journal of Medicine* reported that osteoarthritis can be caused by an inherited genetic abnormality. Experts now believe that at least 25 per cent of all cases of osteoarthritis have a genetic basis. Several teams of researchers are now working to develop gene therapy for the condition.

An ancient disorder

If you think arthritis is mostly a modernday affliction, think again: it is recognized as one of the oldest ailments known to man and beast.

Evidence shows that arthritis has afflicted not only humans for thousands of years but in fact has also affected virtually every animal that has joints. The earliest known signs of arthritis have turned up in the fossilized skeleton of diplodocus, a dinosaur that lived about 60 million years ago. More recently in history, skeletal evidence of osteoarthritis has been found in the remains of

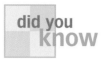

Neanderthal man and in Egyptian mummies. In fact, a 5,300-year-old mummy, nicknamed Oetzi, is believed to have suffered from arthritis, and the numerous tattoos on his body may have been an ancient therapy for his condition.

Through the centuries, arthritis has obviously been an important and widespread human affliction. Artists have long used bent-backed human figures and hands with gnarled fingers to symbolize the frailty of old age. Shakespeare referred to arthritic diseases in *A Midsummer Night's Dream* ('Therefore the moon…/Pale in her anger, washes all the air/That rheumatic diseases do abound'), and John Milton cited them in *Paradise Lost*: 'Disease is a consequence of man's imperfection – dropsies, asthmas, and joint-wracking rheumatism.'

From caveman to modern man

Arthritis remains a widespread affliction today. It is the most common chronic disabling condition in the UK, affecting more people than diabetes. According to estimates from the Arthritis Research Campaign, some 7 million adults in the UK (15 per cent of the population) have long-term health problems as a result of arthritis and related conditions. This figure is expected to rise to almost 10 million by 2020.

The cost of arthritis Arthritis and related conditions are the second most common cause of days off work, accounting for 206 million lost working days in the UK in 1999-2000. Almost 9 million UK patients visited their GP in the past year with arthritis-related problems, and more than 2.8 million of

Arthritis through the ages

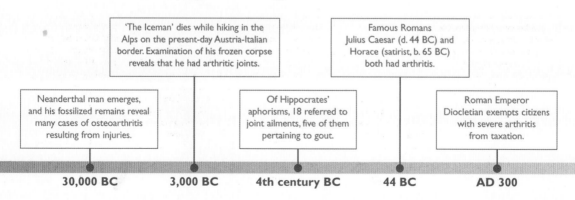

'The Iceman' dies while hiking in the Alps on the present-day Austria-Italian border. Examination of his frozen corpse reveals that he had arthritic joints.

Famous Romans Julius Caesar (d. 44 BC) and Horace (satirist, b. 65 BC) both had arthritis.

Neanderthal man emerges, and his fossilized remains reveal many cases of osteoarthritis resulting from injuries.

Of Hippocrates' aphorisms, 18 referred to joint ailments, five of them pertaining to gout.

Roman Emperor Diocletian exempts citizens with severe arthritis from taxation.

30,000 BC   **3,000 BC**   **4th century BC**   **44 BC**   **AD 300**

Ailments by numbers

The lives of hundreds of thousands of people in the UK are limited by illness and disease. The figures below show the number of people currently estimated to be suffering from the most common types of ailment. For cancer, the statistic reflects diagnosed cases.

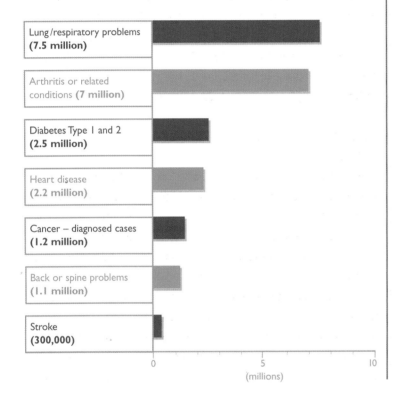

Lung/respiratory problems **(7.5 million)**

Arthritis or related conditions **(7 million)**

Diabetes Type 1 and 2 **(2.5 million)**

Heart disease **(2.2 million)**

Cancer – diagnosed cases **(1.2 million)**

Back or spine problems **(1.1 million)**

Stroke **(300,000)**

0   5   10

(millions)

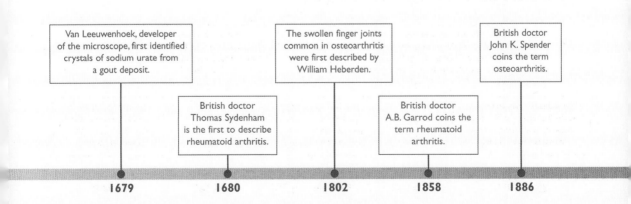

Van Leeuwenhoek, developer of the microscope, first identified crystals of sodium urate from a gout deposit.

British doctor Thomas Sydenham is the first to describe rheumatoid arthritis.

The swollen finger joints common in osteoarthritis were first described by William Heberden.

British doctor A.B. Garrod coins the term rheumatoid arthritis.

British doctor John K. Spender coins the term osteoarthritis.

1679   1680   1802   1858   1886

Survey says?

Adults with arthritis are substantially worse off than others when it comes to health-related quality of life, according to a report from the US Centers for Disease Control and Prevention. Researchers surveyed more than 32,000 Americans in 11 states, 29 percent of whom reported having arthritis. 'Respondents with arthritis reported having fair or poor health approximately three times more often than respondents without arthritis,' said the researchers.

those visits were because of osteoarthritis. The number of people with osteoarthritis has increased in the past 10 years. Arthritis is one of the nation's leading causes of disability: in the UK, more than a million people with arthritis have trouble performing everyday activities such as getting dressed, climbing stairs or getting in and out of bed. In addition, arthritis is the main cause of limited mobility in the elderly.

As grim as the statistics seem, there has been exciting progress in research into the causes of the condition. Osteoarthritis, by far the most common form of arthritis, was considered an inevitable part of ageing. But researchers have recently uncovered a number of causes for osteoarthritis – some of which, such as obesity and joint injury – can be corrected in time to prevent the disease.

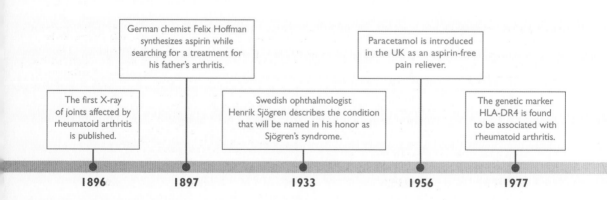

German chemist Felix Hoffman synthesizes aspirin while searching for a treatment for his father's arthritis.

Paracetamol is introduced in the UK as an aspirin-free pain reliever.

The first X-ray of joints affected by rheumatoid arthritis is published.

Swedish ophthalmologist Henrik Sjögren describes the condition that will be named in his honor as Sjögren's syndrome.

The genetic marker HLA-DR4 is found to be associated with rheumatoid arthritis.

1896   1897   1933   1956   1977

> **▶ FACT** Contrary to what many people think, cracking your knuckles doesn't lead to arthritis. The cracking sound is caused by the sudden formation of a gas bubble in the synovial fluid inside the joint. The sound is unpleasant, but the act is harmless.

Exploring oestrogen Women suffer from osteoarthritis more than men, and comprise three-quarters of all cases in the UK. Some researchers have theorized that this correlation is due to the diminishing levels of the female sex hormone, oestrogen, as women age. Scientists already know that lower levels of the hormone at menopause leads to brittle bones and are exploring the relationship between oestrogen and osteoarthritis. Researchers found that women who received supplemental oestrogen for 10 years or longer had a greater reduction in the risk of any hip osteoarthritis as compared with those who took it for less than 10 years. More research is needed, but certainly the oestrogen connection may lead to less suffering for women in future.

Researchers aren't just dwelling on the causes of osteoarthritis; they are also exploring new avenues of treatment for people already suffering long-term aches and pains. Acupuncture, the ancient treatment that has been used to relieve painful conditions for thousands of years, might be potent against osteoarthritis of the knee. A study reported by the University of Maryland, USA, in 1997 suggests that the therapy, when combined with conventional medical therapy, reduces pain in an osteoarthritic knee.

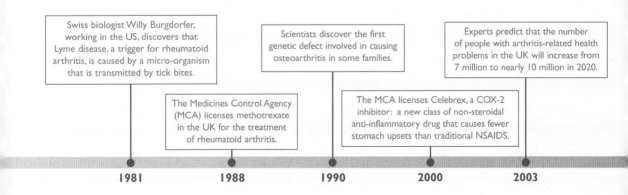

Swiss biologist Willy Burgdorfer, working in the US, discovers that Lyme disease, a trigger for rheumatoid arthritis, is caused by a micro-organism that is transmitted by tick bites.

Scientists discover the first genetic defect involved in causing osteoarthritis in some families.

Experts predict that the number of people with arthritis-related health problems in the UK will increase from 7 million to nearly 10 million in 2020.

The Medicines Control Agency (MCA) licenses methotrexate in the UK for the treatment of rheumatoid arthritis.

The MCA licenses Celebrex, a COX-2 inhibitor: a new class of non-steroidal anti-inflammatory drug that causes fewer stomach upsets than traditional NSAIDS.

1981   1988   1990   2000   2003

> '**I don't think many people realize how large a problem arthritis is. These are big numbers that are going to get a lot bigger.'**
>
> —Sophie Edwards, Chief Executive, ARMA.

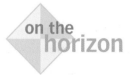

on the horizon

◗ The US National Institutes of Health's National Center for Complementary and Alternative Medicine has begun two clinical trials for the treatment of osteoarthritis. One will test glucosamine and chondroitin sulphate, two of the most promising dietary supplements for treating osteoarthritis. Results are due in 2005. The second trial will evaluate acupuncture for the treatment of pain associated with osteoarthritis. Results are expected in autumn 2003.

Fresh insights into RA Rheumatoid arthritis is also revealing its secrets to researchers, who have found that a protein which occurs naturally – tumour necrosis factor – plays a crucial role in causing joint inflammation and damage. Using genetic engineering, researchers have developed two new drugs, Enbrel and Remi-cade, that block tumour necrosis factor. These and other new 'disease-modifying drugs have revolutionized the treatment of rheumatoid arthritis.

Much talked about these days is mino-cycline, an antibiotic drug from the tetracycline family that was used originally to treat acne. The medication may be able to block enzymes that destroy cartilage inside joints.

In addition, a very promising treatment that may actually cure rheumatoid arthritis was reported in 2000. Further results were announced in 2002, backing up the good work of the first results. Developed by researchers at University College in London, the treatment involves depleting the blood of B lymphocytes; these immune cells form antibodies that cause much of the joint destruction that occurs in rheumatoid arthritis.

Attacking arthritis: the combined support of healthcare specialists

Researchers aren't the only ones trying to get to the bottom of the condition. As there is no national service for musculoskeletal conditions in the UK, the rise of arthritis has galvanized the efforts of the Arthritis and Musculoskeletal Alliance (ARMA) working with the British Society of Rheumatology and various arthritis support groups such as Arthritis Care and the Arthritis Research Campaign. They joined forces in 2003 to determine standards of healthcare to meet the needs of people with arthritis.

Their effort, known as the Standards Care Project, is a two year project and has certain goals, including:

◗ Setting standards for high-quality healthcare for people who suffer from arthritis.

◗ Increasing public awareness of arthritis as the leading cause of disability and an important health problem.

Exorcising pain before exercise

There are known methods of stopping arthritis pain for short periods of time. Here are several methods you can use before exercising or just going out for the groceries:

Moist heat Applying warm towels, hot packs or taking a bath or shower for 15 minutes three times a day can relieve pain.

Cold A bag of ice wrapped in a towel helps to stop pain and reduce swelling when used for 10 to 15 minutes at a time. This is especially effective for inflamed joints.

Relaxation therapy Patients can learn to release the tension in their muscles to relieve pain.

Mobilization therapies Traction (gentle, steady pulling), massage and manipulation (using the hands to restore normal movement to stiff joints) can all help to control pain and increase joint motion and muscle and tendon flexibility.

- Supporting people who suffer from arthritis in developing and accessing the resources they need, in order to manage their condition.

- Supporting service-providers in planning and delivering high-quality arthritis services.

- Ensuring that people with arthritis receive the family, community and peer support they need.

As you can see, the war on arthritis is a all-out effort. But until more progress is made, you will continue to be the architect of how you live with it. You will need to take those first proactive steps that will help you to lead as normal a life as possible. And you can do it with *Taking Charge of Arthritis* by your side. The book gives you everything you require to help you to achieve your goals: guidance in becoming a self-manager of your arthritis as well as the latest information on the pain-relieving treatments that best fit your needs.

did you know

- Switching from high heels to flatties may decrease a woman's chances of developing osteoarthritis. One study claims that women who walk in high-heeled shoes strain the area between the kneecap and the thighbone, especially in the inner side of the joint. This joint-strain may contribute to osteoarthritis.

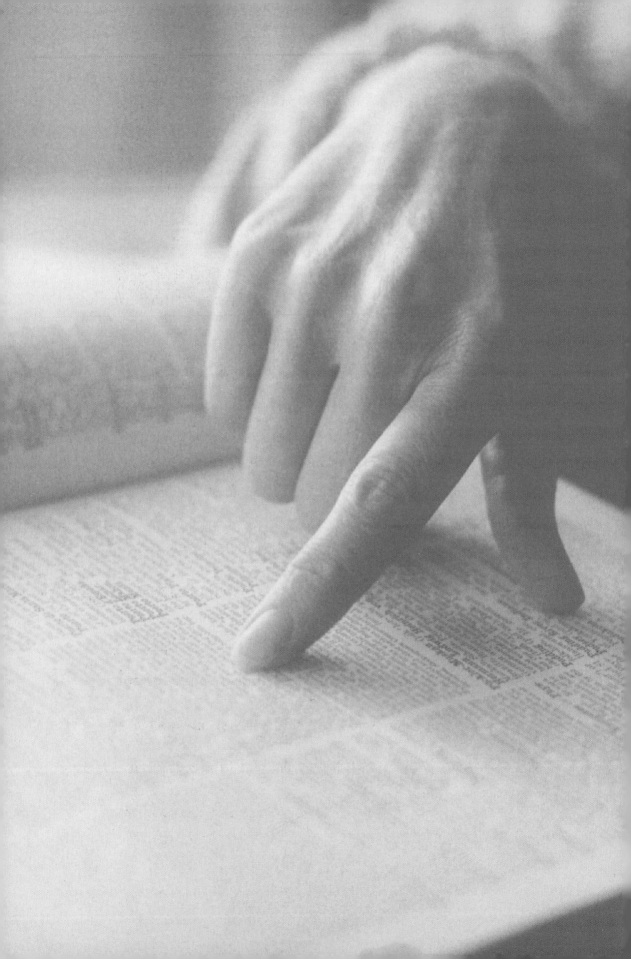

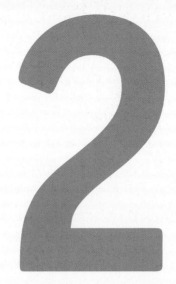

Know your arthritis

Knowing how a healthy body works,

and understanding what goes wrong

when arthritis attacks, can help you to

take control of your own treatment

and pain relief. It will also put you in a

position to make informed decisions

about your own healthcare.

Knowledge is power

Many people suffering with arthritis are caught up in a devastating cycle of pain, depression and stress. Becoming an active participant in managing your pain, however, can break that vicious circle and help you to overcome your personal fear. Knowing what's going on in your body can impose a much-needed sense of calm and enable you to make clear-headed decisions.

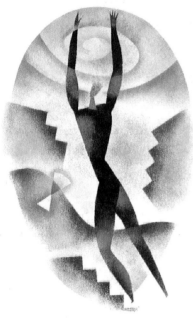

THE MORE YOU KNOW about your particular type of arthritis, the greater your chances of overcoming the pain and the limitations it imposes on you.

An equal-opportunity condition

Arthritis encompasses some 127 different diseases. So when you say, 'I have arthritis,' the logical response is, 'What kind?' Arthritis, in its many forms, can strike all ages and both sexes. Some forms – rheumatoid arthritis, fibromyalgia, and lupus – are more prevalent among women; gout and ankylosing spondylitis are more common in men.

Arthritis has many faces. It may affect only one joint or many of them. You may experience only mild pain while someone else may suffer from excruciating aches and extreme fatigue. You may find that your symptoms will fluctuate between great pain and periods of quiescence while a friend's symptoms may remain stable for years. Some forms of the disease are caused by metabolic disorders, others are due to congenital defects in the joints, and still others may result from environmental factors – what we do or don't eat, for example.

Arthritis basics This chapter will ground you thoroughly in the most common types of arthritis. In each case, we describe the condition and explain its causes and the progression of symptoms. We also provide you with an invaluable insight into how each type of arthritis should be diagnosed, what you should do once you are diagnosed and, of course, the most promising treatments. Later chapters will tell you more about treatments – the exercises, drugs, nutrition, stress-reduction techniques, and alternative approaches that can help you to overcome your arthritis problem. We begin with understanding the anatomy of a joint – the starting point for virtually every type of arthritis.

The feminine side of arthritis

According to the Arthritis Research Campaign, 5.2 million women – but only 3.7 million men – visited a GP for arthritis or related conditions, in 2000. Possible explanations for this discrepancy include women's weaker cartilage and tendons, or a link to the female sex hormone, oestrogen. All remain unproven, but the statistical evidence in the UK underscores women's affliction with the condition. For example:

Osteoarthritis (OA) of the hand affects nearly 3 million women (67 per cent of all cases); OA of the knee affects 440,000 women (80 per cent of all cases); and OA of the hips affects 105,000 women (50 per cent of all cases).

Rheumatoid arthritis affects 282,400 women representing 73 per cent of all cases.

Systemic lupus erythematosus (SLE) affects 9,000-9,500 women, representing about 90 per cent of all cases.

Fibromyalgia affects an estimated 1.2 million Britons; nine out of ten are women.

Juvenile rheumatoid arthritis affects 8,600 girls, representing 71 per cent of all cases.

Bones and joints

Bones are connected to each other at joints, which can be grouped into three classes, based on the amount of movement they allow: fixed joints, slightly movable joints and freely movable joints.

Fixed joints These joints allow no movement whatever. Examples of fixed joints include those separating the bones of the pelvis, which bend only during delivery to ease the baby's movement down the birth canal, and the joints (known as sutures) between the bones of the skull.

Slightly movable joints These joints allow a limited amount of motion. They can be found, for example, in the bones of the spinal column that are held together by tough pads (or 'discs') of fibrocartilage. Usually known as intervertebral joints, they secure the bones tightly, but do provide some flexibility, allowing you to bend and stretch.

Freely movable joints Also known as synovial joints, they usually leap to mind when we think of arthritis. Examples are the hips, knees, elbows, fingers and – most mobile of all – the shoulder joint, whose ball-and-socket structure enables you to move your arm in a complete circle.

Name that joint

You know them by the names elbow, shoulder and knee. But every joint in the body also has a scientific name as well. Take this little anatomical quiz, trying to match each of the numbered joints on the left with its scientific name on the right.

1 Shoulder

2 Knee

3 Wrist

4 Joint that connects a spinal vertebra

5 Joint where spine joins pelvis

6 Joint where ribs join breastbone

7 Finger joint

8 Joint at the base of the thumb

9 Bunion joint at the base of the toe

Ⓐ Sacroiliac

Ⓑ Costochondral joint

Ⓒ First metatarsophalangeal joint

Ⓓ Glenohumeral

Ⓔ Tibiofemoral

Ⓕ Radiocarpal

Ⓖ Facet joint

Ⓗ Interphalangeal joint

Ⓘ First carpometacarpal joint

Answers **1**Ⓓ **2**Ⓔ **3**Ⓕ **4**Ⓖ **5**Ⓐ **6**Ⓑ **7**Ⓗ **8**Ⓘ **9**Ⓒ

○ **FACT** The human skeleton contains more than 200 bones, which are connected by almost 150 joints.

○ By the age of 65, more than half of all people who have been X-rayed show evidence of osteoarthritis in at least one joint.

Joints: how things work

The freely movable joints are the prime location for many types of arthritis, including the two most common – osteoarthritis and rheumatoid arthritis. It is likely that your arthritis affects one or more of your synovial joints, so you need to understand them and have an idea of what is involved in their everyday operation.

Bones

The ends of bones form the heart of a synovial joint. When you bend, twist, or turn, joints provide the flexibility to move these bones into position. Most of our everyday actions – walking, sitting down, washing dishes – require the smooth movement of bones within the joints.

Articular cartilage

This is a rubbery, gel-like tissue that sits at the end of the bones where they meet at a joint. Cartilage provides a smooth surface so that bones can move easily through their range of motion without grating against each other. This smooth movement is aided by the slippery synovial fluid that bathes the joint. Articular (which simply means joint) cartilage also plays a crucial shock-absorbing role.

When you run, for instance, you exert between four and eight times your body's weight on your knees and hips. Even ordinary walking can double the weight on those joints with every step you take. Exercise can stimulate the healthy flow of synovial fluid into and out of the cartilage. When there is no pressure on a joint, synovial fluid flows into the cartilage, bathing it in nutrients needed to strengthen the tissue and maintain its health. When pressure is exerted – when you run or walk, for example – the fluid seeps out

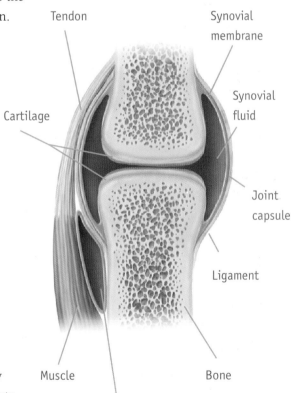

Tendon

Synovial membrane

Synovial fluid

Cartilage

Joint capsule

Ligament

Muscle

Bone

Bursa

Bursitis: cushions in crisis

Small sacs called bursae are found near certain joints, including the elbow and knee. These sacs are filled with synovial fluid and act as cushions, taking the pressure off the surface of a bone or easing the friction created on tendons or muscles when a joint is in motion.

Bursitis – inflammation of one or more bursae – usually occurs when people repeatedly put pressure on a joint. For example, carpet installers, who must kneel for long periods of time, may develop bursitis of the knee. Or students who prop their heads on their elbows when studying may develop 'student's elbow'.

Bursitis or arthritis? Bursitis is a 'local' problem – only the bursae are affected – but is often mistaken for arthritis. The inflammation causes pain, tenderness and, sometimes, swelling; moving the joint often makes the problem worse. Anti-inflammatory drugs such as aspirin or ibuprofen can sometimes help, and so can applying an ice pack. But often the best treatment for bursitis is simply to rest the affected joint, which allows the excess fluid inside the bursa to become reabsorbed into the bloodstream.

of the cartilage, absorbing and dispersing the pressure. Without synovial fluid pulsing through it regularly, cartilage would almost certainly, slowly dry out.

> **◗ FACT** Excess weight hurts. Every extra pound of weight you gain will put 4-8lb more stress and strain onto your knees and hips.

Joint capsule
The bones of the joint are covered by a tough, fibrous covering called the joint capsule. The capsule's outer layer is made of interwoven bands of collagen fibres that provide the joint capsule with strength and flexibility.

Synovial membrane

The joint capsule's inner surface is lined with a delicate layer of tissue called the synovial membrane, which contains cells that produce and release synovial fluid. This clear, yellow, sticky fluid is 95 per cent water, has the consistency of egg white (*synovia* means 'like egg white'), and helps to nourish and lubricate the cartilage and bones within the joint capsule. Aided by the synovial fluid, the cartilage-tipped bones in a healthy joint glide over each other smoothly, creating even less friction than ice sliding on ice.

Ligaments

These strong, flexible bands of tissue help to stabilize the joint by binding together the bones within it. Most ligaments lack elasticity, but some do stretch to allow slight separation of the bones that they connect.

Tendons

Also known as sinews, tendons assist the ligaments in stabilizing and supporting the joints. These strong white cords of fibrous tissue serve to attach muscles to the bones of the joint.

Muscles

Your muscles are the force that moves the bones within a joint, holding the joint ends together and bringing them back into alignment after movement. Even the simplest movement you make requires at least two muscles acting in equal and opposite ways; one muscle contracts and pulls on its attached tendon, which in turn pulls on a bone and moves it. At the same time, the opposing muscle relaxes to allow the movement to occur.

Osteoarthritis: good cartilage gone bad

Osteoarthritis (OA) is by far the most common type of arthritis, affecting hands, knees and hips, in particular. There is no official figure for the number of people suffering from arthritis in Britain, but it is estimated at well over 2 million. Although it is called 'old people's arthritis' or degenerative joint disease, it can affect younger people, too. Whatever your age, OA needs to be approached with an informed strategy.

What is OA?

Since *osteo* is the Greek word for bone, you may have thought that osteoarthritis is a bone disorder. But actually the condition involves mainly cartilage, the protective tissue that covers and cushions the ends of the bones within the joint.

> ◯ **FACT** Osteoarthritis can occur in any joint in the body, but most commonly affects the hips, knees, lower back, neck and fingers. OA in the wrists, elbows and ankles can often be traced to an injury or to an occupation that subjects them to repeated stress.

Dysfunctional cartilage In OA, the cartilage doesn't function as it was intended and, for a variety of reasons, slowly breaks down. A number of possible causes – injury to the cartilage, genetic mutations and factors associated with ageing – can precipitate the breakdown. The result is that the cartilage wears away, which is why osteoarthritis is sometimes referred to as 'wear-and-tear' or 'degenerative' arthritis. As the cartilage erodes, joints no longer move smoothly but instead feel, and sometimes sound, creaky.

Most OA sufferers have what is called primary OA, meaning the cause of their cartilage breakdown isn't known. In cases of secondary OA, cartilage damage can be traced to a specific cause such as a physical injury to the joint, inflammation due to rheumatoid arthritis or to misaligned bones.

Unlike some other types of arthritis, such as rheumatoid arthritis, OA affects only the joints and not any other parts of the body. Not surprisingly, OA is most likely to develop in those joints that are subject to the greatest amount of stress: the body's weight-bearing joints, especially the knees and hips.

Cartilage: the inside story

Water
Articular cartilage is mostly water – 80 per cent, in fact. Its high water content helps cartilage to cushion the bones from trauma. Cartilage derives its water from the synovial fluid that bathes and lubricates the bones in a joint.

Collagen
This protein comes in the form of rod-shaped fibres that are the main building block for skin, tendons, bones and other connective tissues. As a key ingredient in cartilage, collagen strengthens cartilage and helps it to resist being pulled apart by pressure or other traumas.

Proteoglycans
Cartilage owes its high water content to proteoglycans. These are molecules that have the unique ability to soak up and hold fluid in the cartilage, allowing it to flow in and out as pressure on a joint increases and decreases. Strands of proteoglycans team up with collagen to form a web-like, water-filled matrix that provides cartilage with its sponge-like resilience, its ability to absorb pressure, and its surface slickness. OA begins with the breakdown of this matrix of proteoglycans and collagen.

Chondrocytes
Scattered throughout cartilage, these cartilage-producing cells are responsible for synthesizing and repairing the cartilage 'scaffolding' – namely, its collagen and proteoglycan molecules.

The road to osteoarthritis As cartilage breaks down, it no longer cushions bones or prevents them from rubbing against each other. In addition, bony swellings or spurs (known as osteophytes) may develop around the edge of bones in response to pressure on them. These changes lead to pain, stiffness and a restricted range of motion.

What causes OA?

The cause of primary osteoarthritis – what triggers joint cartilage to erode – is not known. The disease process apparently begins when destructive enzymes damage the network of collagen fibres that maintain the structure of cartilage. With its collagen 'super-structure' damaged, cartilage swells with water, becoming softer and more vulnerable to stresses that wear it away. Researchers have identified several risk factors that can significantly increase a person's odds of developing the disease.

Debunking cartilage myths

Until recently, osteoarthritis was wrongly viewed as a natural consequence of getting older – an inevitable result of decades of wear and tear on the joints. But scientists studying cartilage have made some exciting discoveries suggesting that the cartilage breakdown leading to osteoarthritis is by no means inevitable.

Once considered simple and inert, cartilage is living tissue. A hotbed of metabolic activity, cartilage is constantly being both produced and broken down. In fact, a dietary supplement, chondroitin sulphate, may help to rebuild cartilage by suppressing enzymes that destroy cartilage. Drugs that may achieve the same result are now being studied.

In one significant study, researchers analysed joint cartilage from elderly people with osteoarthritis and from people of the same age who were free of the disease, and found some striking differences. Compared with cartilage from disease-free people, cartilage from patients with osteoarthritis contained more water (making cartilage softer and more fragile), higher levels of cartilage-destroying enzymes, and smaller amounts of proteoglycans, the molecules so vital for cartilage resilience.

The dietary supplement glucosamine may work against osteoarthritis, and perhaps even help to prevent it, by replenishing the proteoglycans inside cartilage.

Healthy joint

Arthritic joint

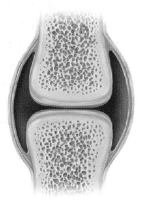
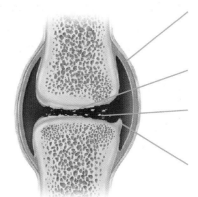

Thickened synovial membrane

Worn-away cartilage

Cartilage fragments in synovial fluid

Bone spur

In a healthy joint (left), the bones are capped by smooth cartilage. The surrounding joint capsule has an inner lining that produces synovial fluid, which helps to lubricate the joint. In a joint with osteoarthritis (right), the cartilage has become roughened and partially worn away. Chunks of broken-off cartilage have irritated the synovial membrane, making it inflamed and thickened. Loss of cartilage has increased pressure on the bones, which have formed spurs, known as osteophytes, around their edges.

◉ **FACT** If you have arthritis, there is a scientific name – crepitus – for the creaky feeling (and creaky noises) that you may notice when you move affected joints. Doctors feel and listen for signs of crepitus when diagnosing arthritis in patients.

Age

Clearly the most powerful predictor of whether a person will develops osteoarthritis, is the individual's age. The condition is rare in young people, but becomes increasingly more common in older age groups. However, don't misunderstand the facts: osteoarthritis may correlate with age, but it isn't caused by it.

Instead, it now appears that factors associated with ageing – and, indeed, quite a few other factors as well – can make people susceptible to OA and cause their condition to worsen.

on the horizon

◉ As they seek the underlying cause of osteoarthritis, researchers are expanding their search beyond cartilage and into the underlying bone. Accumulating evidence suggests that changes in bone 'turnover' – the counterbalancing process of bone synthesis and bone breakdown – may be involved in causing osteoarthritis. 'Indeed, the cartilage may be the innocent bystander in a disease process that is centred more in bone than in cartilage,' writes researcher Paul Dieppe of the Department of Social Medicine at Bristol University.

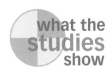

what the **studies** show

▶ A study of former American footballers found that more than 80 per cent of players with a history of a knee injury had evidence of osteoarthritis 10 to 30 years after their careers had ended.

Too many pounds

Wisdom isn't the only thing that increases with age: so does the waistline. Carrying around extra pounds puts constant stress on the joints that will eventually damage the cartilage. This is particularly true for the weight-bearing joints: the knees and, to a lesser extent, the hips.

If you're overweight, losing those pounds is one of the most effective of all osteoarthritis treatments available. A study that followed women of different weights over 36 years found that the heaviest women (those in the upper 20 per cent by weight) were more than three times more likely than women in the bottom 20 per cent to develop severe osteoarthritis of the knee. This was the first study showing that OA may be prevented.

Loose joints

When the bones of a joint aren't bound tightly to each other, they can bang together and damage their protective cartilage. Such 'joint instability' is now recognized as a major cause of the pain and early morning stiffness that may occur long before cartilage damage has begun. (Such symptoms are often felt by young, 'double-jointed' women whose flexibility makes them talented ballet dancers.) As a preventive measure, people with loose joints may be advised to avoid activities that could increase their risk of developing osteoarthritis prematurely.

On-the-job exertion

Certain jobs increase a person's risk of developing osteoarthritis. For example, OA of the knee is common among miners, dock-workers, and others who must constantly bend their knees or do heavy lifting on the job.

Look to your genes

In 1990, after studying a family whose members developed osteoarthritis in many of their joints at a very early age, researchers reported that they had traced osteoarthritis to a gene responsible for making the collagen in cartilage. A mutation in this gene causes defective collagen to be produced, which probably weakens cartilage and causes it to break down prematurely.

Genes seem to influence osteoarthritis in particular joints as well. In 1944, researchers reported that OA involving the end joints of the fingers was an inherited trait. In this condition, small bony knobs known as Heberden's nodes (named after the 18th-century British physician who first described them) form on the top of the finger joints. Heberden's nodes are more common in women, particularly after menopause.

Genes may also influence OA in other joints. In 1998, researchers who were studying 616 pairs of identical and fraternal female twins aged over 40 concluded that genetic factors may be responsible for half of all cases of OA of the hip.

Arthritis profile

Mike Atherton

In August 1990, instead of celebrating the century he had scored in front of his home crowd against India – the highlight of his test career up to then – Mike Atherton was experiencing terrible pain in his buttocks and down his legs. Shortly afterwards, X-rays showed a stress-fracture in his lower back. In August 1991 he had an operation to repair the fracture and although he followed a three-month rehabilitation programme, the pain and stiffness did not go away. More scans were done, and this time two dark and blurred lines were seen and ankylosing spondylitis (AS) was diagnosed. AS (see page 78) is a form of arthritis causing chronic inflammation of the spine, and the former England cricket captain had inherited the condition from his father.

Atherton took Voltarol for many years, but this anti-inflammatory can produce side effects. By the end of his final series as a Test player, Atherton was caught up in a vicious circle of taking bigger doses of Voltarol to get through games, which then caused colitis to flare up. Finally, having had to resort to cortisone injections to cope with the pain, he retired from cricket, aged only 33.

Despite his arthritis, since making his Test debut in 1989, Mike Atherton played 115 Test matches. When he bowed out at the Oval, he ended his international career as the leading English run-scorer in Test cricket since January 1990.

Can you run away from osteoarthritis?

If repetitive stresses can lead to osteoarthritis, are recreational runners at risk? Numerous studies have tried to answer this question, with decidedly mixed results.

For and against A 1996 study looked for signs of osteoarthritis in a group of former top female athletes (middle and long-distance runners and tennis players) and in a control group of women of the same age from the general population. The ex-athletes were two to three times more likely than women in the control group to have osteoarthritis of the knees and hips. And a study published in 2000 found that men under 50 who regularly run more than 20 miles a week faced an increased risk of osteoarthritis of the knee or hip.

But other studies, involving amateur and recreational runners, have found no link between running and osteoarthritis. One study, comparing 17 male runners who had run an average of 28 miles a week for 12 years with non-running men the same average weight and age (56 years old), found no differences in osteoarthritis prevalence between the two groups.

'Joints aren't like the bearings on your car, which wear out after a certain number of miles,' said Dr. Joseph Buckwalter, in his 1998 review of the often-conflicting literature on athletics and osteoarthritis. 'Using the joints doesn't necessarily hurt them – in fact, the more you use them, the better off you may be.'

Bottom line The consensus among experts is that recreational running or other high-impact exercise may accelerate osteoarthritis in previously damaged joints or when done strenuously for a number of years. Runners with healthy joints have less cause for worry, but probably shouldn't overdo it.

Being a woman doesn't help

Women stand a much greater chance of developing osteoarthritis than men, especially as they get older. This gender difference is most extreme for OA of the knee in older people: Women over 65 are more than twice as likely to develop it as men the same age.

Couch potatoes beware

People tend to exercise less as they age – especially if they have arthritis. What's less well appreciated is that inactivity itself increases your risk of osteoarthritis in several ways:

- ● Inactivity leads to weight gain that puts extra strain on the joints – 4-8lb more stress for every extra pound gained.

- ● Tissues vital to joint movement – especially the muscles – can atrophy as a result of inactivity. Studies have shown that people with weak thigh muscles are more likely to develop OA of the knee.

- ● Inactivity can kill off chondrocytes, the cells that make and repair cartilage. Because cartilage has no blood vessels, chondrocytes must obtain nutrients from the synovial fluid. Walking or other weight-bearing activities contract and expand cartilage with each repetition, creating the pumping action of fluid vital for chondrocytes.

Taking a blow

The sports pages regularly report on athletes who've sustained serious injury to a joint – most often the knee. Unfortunately, an athlete or anyone else who suffers an injury to some part of

caution

Early diagnosis and treatment is the best approach for any type of osteoarthritis, but is especially important for osteoarthritis of the knee. Treatment, which may include taking certain drugs, undergoing a weight-loss programme, doing specific exercises, a course of injections of hyaluronic acid and using walking aids, can all help to prevent further joint damage. If left untreated, osteoarthritis of the knee can become disabling, with joint replacement surgery the only recourse for a patient.

Do you have osteoarthritis? Review your symptoms

▶ One or more joints has a deep and aching pain that is steady or intermittent

▶ Pain is worsened by exercise or other activities and eased by rest

▶ Joint pain develops and won't go away, even after resting the joint for several days

▶ One or more joints feel stiff for 30 minutes or less after you get out of bed

▶ One or more joints swell or feel tender

▶ Affected joint has grinding feeling or makes a grinding sound

▶ When you start moving after sitting during the day – after driving a fairly long distance or watching television, for example – you feel stiff for the next 20 or 30 minutes

a joint – such as cartilage, bone, ligament, or tendon – may eventually develop osteoarthritis in that joint. Unfortunately, with some injuries, such as a compound fracture of the ankle, osteoarthritis is almost a certainty. Many professional athletes who incur frequent knee injuries will develop osteoarthritis of the knee after their playing days are over.

The joints that OA targets

Osteoarthritis can affect any of the body's joints, but it most often occurs in the hands, knees, hips or spine.

Hands Osteoarthritis of the fingers is usually hereditary. Heberden's nodes, the small bony knobs that form on the ends of finger joints, occur most often in middle-aged and older women. The nodes are usually painless and tend to develop so slowly over many years that a woman may not notice them until, for example, she has trouble slipping a ring over the joint. These unsightly nodes are twice as likely to develop in women whose mothers also have them. Similar enlargements on the middle finger joints are known as Bouchard's nodes. Both Heberden's and Bouchard's nodes may first develop in one or a few fingers and later affect others. As Heberden himself noted, the problem with these nodes is mainly cosmetic.

A more painful form of OA affecting the end joints of fingers is called nodal osteoarthritis. A single joint suddenly becomes painful, tender, and swollen for three or four weeks, and then the problem subsides. Nodal OA is also hereditary and mainly affects women 45 and older, who are ten times more likely to develop it than men in the same age group.

The joint at the base of the thumb also commonly develops osteoarthritis. By contrast, OA rarely affects the knuckles (where the fingers attach to the palm of the hand).

Knees The knees bear more weight than any other joint in the body, which makes them very susceptible to OA. When that happens, your knees may become swollen and feel stiff and painful when you try to move them. You may notice you have trouble walking, climbing stairs and getting in and out of the car. According to studies, strengthening the muscles surrounding the knee can often dramatically improve the symptoms of osteoarthritis of the knee.

> **caution**
>
> Joint pain that does not abate after a few days of rest is a clear signal that you should see a doctor soon.

Hips Like the knees, the hips are weight-bearing joints and are similarly susceptible to osteoarthritis. People with osteoarthritis of the hip may have trouble bending, and the pain and stiffness may cause them to limp when they walk. The pain may not only be felt in the hip but may also radiate to other parts of the body, especially the groin or down the inside of the thigh.

As we've already said, some cases of osteoarthritis of the hip seem to be hereditary. Also, people who are bow-legged or who have other congenital abnormalities that may have caused the bones of the hip to become misaligned are at increased risk of hip osteoarthritis.

Losing weight can help, but is not as helpful for relieving hip osteoarthritis as it is for the knee. Drugs and exercise can also help to relieve pain and improve movement. Hip-replacement surgery is very effective when other treatments fall short of relieving the pain or disability.

Spine Osteoarthritis of the spine mainly causes stiffness and pain in the neck or in the lower back. Measures that can help to relieve the symptoms include exercises that strengthen the muscles of the back and abdomen, heat treatments and the use of support pillows when sitting. In some people, bone spurs growing from the edges of the vertebrae may squeeze the spinal nerves, causing pain, weakness or numbness in the arms or legs. When this happens, surgery may be necessary to relieve the pressure on the nerves.

How does OA progress?

The breakdown of cartilage that leads to OA doesn't occur overnight, although that first sharp pain in your hip or knee may make you think it does. This erosion almost always occurs slowly, over many months or years, as the once-smooth and slippery cartilage becomes thinner, develops a roughened surface, and loses its cushioning ability.

> 'Joints aren't like the bearings on your car, which wear out after a certain number of miles. The more you use them, the better off you may be.'
>
> — Dr. Joseph Buckwalter, Iowa University, USA

In the same way, the pain and stiffness that accompany the disintegrating cartilage may appear so gradually that many people ignore it or put it down to 'getting older.' And for many lucky people, this is as far as osteoarthritis ever progresses: It remains a mild problem, causing symptoms of which they're barely aware.

When cartilage continues eroding, however, people may begin experiencing the niggling symptoms that eventually send them to the doctor's surgery. After exercise, knees and other joints may ache or feel stiff for a brief time. You may also feel stiff after you've been sitting for a while – when climbing out of the car after a long ride, for example, or getting up after watching a film on TV.

Bone meets bone Eventually, cartilage wears away to the point that, in some areas, bone rubs against bone. People may feel their knees briefly 'lock' as they climb stairs or may feel a grinding sensation – or even hear a grinding sound – when they bend the affected knees or hips. People may also find themselves avoiding once-routine activities that now cause pain – the daily walk to the newsagent, for example, or working in the garden at weekends. If the affected joint is a hip or knee, people may begin to limp as they try to minimize the pain.

Small chunks of fragmented cartilage floating in the synovial fluid may be irritating the synovial membrane and adding to the discomfort; in response, the membrane becomes inflamed, painful, and abnormally thick, and produces excess fluid that makes the joint swell. In addition to pain, a person may now notice that the joint's range of movement has started to become restricted.

Bone spurs and other painful growths OA becomes more severe as changes extend beyond cartilage to the underlying bones, which may sprout small growths (known as bone spurs or osteophytes) around their outer edges. Bone spurs increase the joint's surface area and may be the bones' defensive reaction to the extra pressure created when their protective covering has worn away.

Unfortunately, bone spurs often make things worse: spurs on the spine, for example, may cause severe pain by pinching nerves connecting the spinal cord to the muscles, and sharp spurs that form around the rim of the knee joint may worsen the pain and tenderness. By this time, people may find that arthritis pain is keeping them awake at night.

When cartilage is completely eroded, the sensitive bones rub against each other within the joint. At this point, the pain from osteoarthritis can be excruciating and nearly unrelenting even after the slightest movement. When such severe osteoarthritis affects the weight-bearing joints – the knees or the hips – it can be crippling, especially if:

- ◗ Uneven cartilage loss has created uneven joint surfaces, which causes bones to become misaligned and leads to instability in the joint itself.

- ◗ Extensive bone-spur formation limits a joint's mobility.

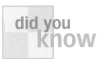

did you know

◗ Osteoarthritis pain tends to worsen towards the end of the day. In many other types of arthritis, pain remains constant during the day or is worse in the morning.

○ Because of lack of use, muscles and tendons that support the joint have shortened and weakened, leading to muscle spasms and more disability. Joint-replacement operations can be a godsend for people with such severe osteoarthritis.

How is OA diagnosed?

Relief for your pain means getting your health problem diagnosed accurately so that treatment can begin. Telling whether you have the disease usually isn't difficult for your doctor. The diagnosis is based on taking details of your clinical history, doing a physical examination and running some tests.

Clinical history

The doctor will ask you a series of questions to get information about your symptoms: when they started, when and where they occur, what they feel like, whether they've changed over

Helping your doctor to get it right

Taking your medical history at the initial visit is a crucial part of the diagnostic process, since it can help your doctor to determine what type of arthritis you have and choose the right laboratory tests to confirm the diagnosis. You can do your doctor and yourself a favour by arriving well prepared. Try to bring with you:

○ A list of other medical problems that you have.

○ A list of all the drugs you take – prescription and over-the-counter as well as herbs or other dietary supplements.

○ A written description of your problem, including: how long ago the joint pain began, whether the symptoms came on suddenly or slowly, which joints were initially affected, what triggered the symptoms (for example, exercise, climbing stairs) and the activities that you can no longer enjoy because joint pain interferes with them.

time, and how they're affecting your life. The doctor will also ask about other diseases from which you may be suffering (and which could also be the cause of your symptoms) and any drugs that you may be taking at the moment (which might interfere with anti-arthritis drugs that may be recommended).

Doctors have found that answers to three questions in particular provide a good gauge of whether a patient has arthritis or some other musculoskeletal disease and how severely disabled he or she is:

> ● Are you experiencing any pain or stiffness in your muscles, joints or back?

> ● Do you ever have any difficulty dressing yourself?

> ● Do you ever have any difficulty walking up and down stairs?

The doctor should then follow up any positive answers with more specific questions. The discussion should also cover:

> ● **Pain** The location of the pain, its severity, character, timing.

> ● **Stiffness** No other condition causes the same type of joint stiffness as osteoarthritis.

> ● **Swelling** At least 85-90 per cent of people with OA don't experience swelling. However, swelling can indicate the degree of joint damage or even suggest that there may be another problem.

> ● **Severity** The degree of pain suggests joint damage and how much treatment you may need.

> ● **Causes** Knowing whether you suffered an injury before the pain started is a valuable clue, which enables the doctor to determine whether you are suffering from secondary OA. If no injury has occurred in the past, it is more likely that your present disorder is primary osteoarthritis.

The physical examination

Following a routine examination to assess your overall health (taking your blood pressure, listening to your heart), the doctor will focus on the joints that are bothering you – feeling and pressing on them for any signs of swelling or tenderness and watching how they 'work' when you walk or bend. The doctor will also assess other joints, which could be affected by arthritis even though you don't know it yet.

During the joint examination, you will be asked to move your joints ('active motion') and the doctor will also move them ('passive motion'). In true joint disease, movement is limited and causes pain with both active and passive motion. If the doctor can move a joint further than you can (flex your knee in a wider arc, for example), then you probably don't have a problem with your joint but instead with the tendons or muscles surrounding it.

Different joints are examined in different ways:

Hands The doctor checks for bony enlargements on the end joints of fingers or on the middle joints. These outgrowths, or nodes, are clear signs of osteoarthritis.

Hips Limited range of motion is the key indicator. With the patient lying on his back with knees bent, the doctor places one hand on the knee and the other on the heel and then rotates the foot outward and inward. Restricted inward rotation is typically an early sign of hip osteoarthritis.

Knees In addition to checking for abnormalities in joint movement, the doctor looks for areas of swelling around the knee joint.

Spine The doctor feels the contours of the spine to check for abnormal tenderness and assesses range of motion – whether the patient can touch his ear with his shoulder, for example.

Laboratory tests

Blood tests Osteoarthritis can almost always be diagnosed without the need for laboratory tests, which are routinely normal in osteoarthritis patients. The main reason for laboratory tests is to rule out the possibility of other diseases such as rheumatoid arthritis. For this reason, some doctors routinely order two blood tests for all patients with painful joints: the rheumatoid factor test and erythrocyte sedimentation. These tests, discussed in more detail on pages 66-67, can help to indicate whether rheumatoid arthritis is present.

Analysing joint fluid Taking a sample of synovial fluid, removed from the joint with a needle, also helps to rule out other possible health problems. Abnormally high levels of white blood cells indicate inflammation and the presence of several possible conditions, including gout, inflammatory types of arthritis such as rheumatoid arthritis or psoriatic arthritis, or arthritis due to an infection (septic arthritis). However, draining fluid from a joint can help to relieve pressure and pain in a joint.

X-rays

These aren't really useful in diagnosing osteoarthritis, since a significant amount of cartilage must be lost before the damage shows up on an X-ray. But X-rays in someone known to have osteoarthritis can reveal the extent of the damage. They can show how much cartilage has been lost, whether underlying bone has been damaged, or whether bone spurs are present. In addition, X-rays taken periodically can monitor the progression of osteoarthritis.

Strange but true Interestingly, the severity of a person's symptoms may be totally unrelated to how the joint looks on an X-ray. In fact, only a third of people whose X-rays show the presence of osteoarthritis, report pain or any other symptoms. On the other hand, some people whose joints look perfectly normal on an X-ray may have excruciating symptoms from osteoarthritis.

Another imaging technique – magnetic resonance imaging, or MRI – excels at revealing injuries to soft tissues such as muscles and tendons. But so far, MRI has no advantage over X-rays in evaluating or monitoring joints affected by osteoarthritis.

What now?

Learning that you have a chronic disease can be disturbing, and a diagnosis of osteoarthritis is no exception. Are you destined for a life of constant pain? Can you continue working, travelling, playing with your grandchildren, or otherwise living life like before? The answers are largely reassuring: OA is not a disease that you need to dread.

The good news Even when it is severe, osteoarthritis is limited to the joints and won't affect your heart, brain or other parts of the body. And today, the great majority of people with OA can be effectively treated – their pain and stiffness eased and

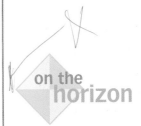

on the horizon

A new procedure developed in Sweden involves removing a sample of healthy cartilage and sending it to a laboratory for cultivation. When millions of cells have grown, surgeons remove the damaged cartilage and replace it with laboratory-grown cartilage. Newer still is an operation in which a small amount of cartilage and bone is removed from the leg, ground up, and placed in the damaged joint, where it stimulates cartilage growth. Clinical trials are soon to take place in the UK, with a review date planned for late 2003.

their joint movement improved – with a combination of anti-inflammatory drugs, exercise, rest, moist heat and the take-charge approach to arthritis described in this book.

Surgical solutions When pain and immobility from hip or knee osteoarthritis can't be relieved in any other way, surgical joint replacement may be necessary. Fortunately, over the past 20 years, medical science has made great advances in joint-replacement surgery, and most people with severe arthritis can look forward to dramatic improvements after undergoing it – free of pain and able to function nearly as well as they did before their osteoarthritis developed.

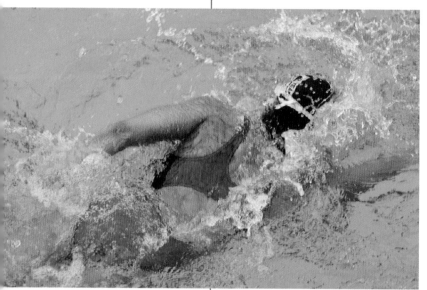

How is OA treated?

There's no need to let arthritis take charge of your life. Instead, you have the power to take charge of it. Virtually all cases of osteoarthritis respond to treatments to ease your pain and stiffness, keep you active and productive, protect and strengthen affected joints, and prevent symptoms from worsening.

To achieve those results, you and your doctor will need to work together, taking into consideration the severity of your symptoms, the joints that are affected, your age, the limitations on your daily activities and other health problems you may have. For many people, a carefully designed combination of several of the following therapies works best. All of them will be discussed more fully in later chapters.

Lose it

Being overweight puts extra stress on your weight-bearing joints – especially your knees and hips. If you're overweight and have osteoarthritis, losing those extra pounds could dramatically improve your symptoms. A sensible diet, that produces steady, sustainable weight-loss is ideal.

Heat it up, or cool it down

Heat applied with a hot-water bottle, hot towels, hot packs, a hot shower or a heating pad can be a very effective treatment for the pain and stiffness of osteoarthritis. For unknown reasons, moist heat seems to provide the greatest relief. Heat can also be administered as either deep or penetrating heat in clinical procedures that use diathermy or ultrasound devices. Cold is most useful for joints that are acutely inflamed – which is rarely a problem in osteoarthritis.

Move it

There was a time when doctors advised their osteoarthritis patients against exercising, believing that exercise could further damage their joints. But research over the past decade has found that exercise ranks as one of the best treatments for OA. The proper exercises can relieve pain, improve flexibility and help you in your weight-loss efforts. As a bonus, exercising will enhance your overall health by reducing stress and lowering your risk of heart disease, diabetes and several types of cancer.

Swallow it

A wide variety of drugs, both over-the-counter and prescription, can help to ease the painful symptoms of osteoarthritis. They include the pain reliever paracetamol, topical or rub-on pain relievers (especially useful for the knee and fingers), and non-steroidal anti-inflammatory drugs (NSAIDs) such as ibuprofen. The NSAIDs relieve pain as well as any inflammation that may be present. Three recently approved NSAIDs – Celebrex, Vioxx, and Mobic – are much less likely to cause bleeding and other gastrointestinal side effects.

Hyaluronic acid injections

People with osteoarthritis of the knee who haven't been helped by NSAIDs or other pain relievers have a new treatment option: injections of hyaluronic acid, a natural substance found in synovial fluid that helps to lubricate the joint. The procedure is called visco-supplementation. The jelly-like hyaluronic acid is injected weekly into the knee for three to five weeks. In clinical

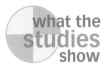

what the studies show

In one animal study, something called cartilage growth factor was combined with fibrinogen, which acts as a glue to hold the growth factor to damaged cartilage. Various concentrations of this mixture were inserted into the joints of several groups of animals. A year later the animals had formed new cartilage.

caution

All NSAIDs are basically equal in effectiveness, but in practice, osteoarthritis patients can respond poorly to one and very well to another. You may have to try several before finding the one that works best for you.

studies, these injections have proved as effective as continual NSAID therapy in providing pain relief that can last for months.

Injected steroids

Injecting steroids directly into a painful joint can temporarily relieve pain and inflammation. Steroids are generally prescribed for an intense flare-up of pain and inflammation or if a patient

Rheumatism: gone but not forgotten

The word *rheumatism* isn't used much anymore, but its origins can be traced back to the ancient Greek theory of disease.

Until about 100 years ago, what we now know as arthritis was mainly referred to as *rheumatism*, a word probably coined in the second century AD by Galen, the illustrious Greek physician. The Greeks believed that diseases were caused by four primary substances, or humours, that flowed from the brain to various parts of the body.

Diseases occurred at the places in the body where these flows stopped. The Greek word *rheuma* means flux and referred to the slow-flowing humour that afflicted the joints and caused pain, swelling and stiffness. Through the centuries that followed, *rheumatism* became a broadly used term for aches and pains anywhere in the body.

Today, doctors rarely call a patient's problem *rheumatism*, but instead diagnose it as a particular type of arthritis. Nevertheless, *rheuma* remains firmly entrenched in arthritis terminology. Rheumatology was created in 1949 as the medical speciality for the study of joint diseases, and its practitioners are rheumatologists; *The Journal of Rheumatology* is a leading publication for highlighting studies on joint diseases; rheumatoid arthritis is a well-known type of arthritis; and an important class of drugs for treating RA is the disease-modifying anti-rheumatic drugs or DMARDs.

doesn't find relief from other painkillers. This short-term measure should not be done more than two or three times a year because of the risk of side effects.

Surgery

Surgeons can make small repairs to cartilage with an arthroscope – a long viewing tube inserted through small incisions in the skin. Arthroscopy can help to alleviate the symptoms of osteoarthritis, but unfortunately it cannot stop the progression of the disease.

Surgery can also help osteoarthritis by preventing the joint from becoming deformed or even by correcting an existing deformity; removing part of the bone around the joint to allow for movement; replacing a damaged joint with an artificial joint made of plastic, metal or ceramic; or immobilizing a joint to correct severe joint problems.

Alternative treatments

Several dietary supplements (glucosamine, chondroitin sulphate and SAM-e) show promise in osteoarthritis treatment, not only for relieving pain but also for rebuilding cartilage. In addition, studies show that adequate intake of vitamins including C, E and beta carotene may reduce your risk of developing osteoarthritis or, if you already have it, prevent it from worsening.

Rheumatoid arthritis: fire in the joints

Rheumatoid arthritis (RA) is the most common type of inflammatory arthritis and usually affects many joints in the body. RA is much less common than osteoarthritis, affecting only about 1-3 per cent of the total UK population, or some 387,000 people. Some 1,200 new cases of RA are diagnosed every year, with women accounting for three out of every four people with the disease. RA can begin at any age, but most commonly develops in the middle years – from 30 to 50.

RA versus OA: comparisons and contrasts

Age of occurrence Rheumatoid arthritis (RA) usually develops between the ages of 30 and 50, but can occur at any age. Osteoarthritis (OA) is a disease of middle and old age and rarely occurs before the age of 45.

Pattern of disease RA often strikes symmetrically, meaning it affects both wrists, the knuckles on both hands, etc. OA rarely affects both joints (for example, both wrists) at once.

Speed of onset About 20 per cent of RA cases develop suddenly, within weeks or months. OA develops slowly, with cartilage breakdown usually occurring over several years.

Extent of illness In addition to causing joint damage, RA can cause fatigue, fever, anaemia and weight loss and can damage the heart and other organs. OA is limited to the joints.

Joints affected RA usually affects many joints, including the wrists (affected in almost all RA patients), knuckles, elbows, shoulders, ankles, feet and neck (but usually spares the rest of the spine). OA most commonly affects the knees, hips, feet, hands and spine. It sometimes affects the knuckles and wrists, but rarely affects the elbows and shoulders.

Hand involvement RA affects many of the hand joints, but usually not the end joints closest to the fingertips. OA affects the knuckles closest to the fingertips more often than other joints of the hand.

Morning stiffness People with RA have prolonged morning stiffness, usually lasting for at least 30 minutes after they get up. With OA, morning stiffness lasts for less than 30 minutes.

What is RA?

RA is a systemic disease, meaning it can affect not only the joints but also the blood vessels, heart, skin, muscles and other parts of the body. Most people with RA must contend with daily pain and stiffness that may wax and wane. They often speak of having good and bad days, weeks, or months, and of enduring periods of depression, anxiety and helplessness. The self-empowerment approach suggested throughout this book has proved its usefulness in helping people with RA to gain control over their disease and over their lives.

> ● **FACT** If you have arthritis, you may swear that your stiffness and pain get worse when the weather changes. They probably do. Studies using climate chambers have found that people with arthritis really do experience increased stiffness and pain when the barometric pressure drops quickly or when the humidity suddenly rises.

Do you really have it? Rheumatoid arthritis and osteoarthritis are often mistaken for each other – which can cause serious problems, since the two types of arthritis are treated quite differently. Although symptoms may be similar, RA and OA are very different diseases.

Osteoarthritis can affect any joint that has cartilage – freely movable joints such as the knee or slightly movable joints like the vertebrae. By contrast, RA focuses on the body's freely movable joints and on one area in particular: the synovial membrane, which is the inner lining of the capsule surrounding freely movable joints. Once this joint becomes inflamed, the characteristic symptoms of rheumatoid arthritis – heat, swelling, stiffness and pain – can then be felt.

While osteoarthritis confines its damage to the joints, RA is a systemic disease that can damage not only the joints but also other parts of the body such as blood vessels, the eyes and the heart. This tissue damage is caused by chronic inflammation – the hallmark of RA. Although inflammation can also occur in osteoarthritis, it is confined to the affected joints.

What causes RA?

The causes of RA's key feature – chronic inflammation – are not known. However, scientists do know that a glitch in the immune system is involved. Like psoriasis, lupus, multiple sclerosis and

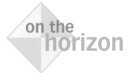

on the **horizon**

● A treatment that may actually cure rheumatoid arthritis was first reported in 2000, and followed up in 2002. Developed by researchers at University College in London, the new treatment involves depleting the blood of B lymphocytes; these immune cells form antibodies that cause much of the joint destruction that occurs in RA. It still needs to be shown that this treatment is safe, but Dr Tom Palfreman of the British Society for Rheumatology says 'B-lymphocyte depletion promises to be a new way of treating RA. The results, to date, show a magnitude of response in patients that exceeds any other therapies currently used'.

continued on page 62

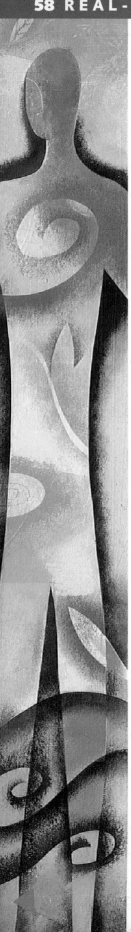

Coping with changes

At 16, Stephen Maguire from Strabane in Northern Ireland became an Irish record-holder for the long jump. A record which remains unbroken, 23 years later. As an international athlete with huge potential at junior level, Stephen was very fit and very focused on his sport.

'But when I was 18, I picked up my first series of injuries. The doctors couldn't get to the bottom of it – why they were being caused. I would pull my hamstring from sneezing – literally!' says Stephen.

Stephen battled against injury, up to the age of 22; every time he got to a certain level of fitness, his body broke down again and, each time, he couldn't get back up again to the same level. 'I would manage to get in a couple of months' training, and was still relatively successful, but I just couldn't get back to the level I was used to, the level I wanted,' Stephen remembers.

'Then, when I was 28, I woke up one morning and couldn't move. I was in severe pain, the right-hand side of my body was badly swollen and I had a red rash. I went straight to see the doctor, who gave me a blood test.'

Rheumatoid arthritis was diagnosed and Stephen had to spend three weeks in hospital, going through various tests and being held under observation. After his spell in hospital, Stephen had to visit the rheumatologist every six weeks, for about six months, just for a check-up and to get to the bottom of what was going on. 'I continued to vomit and suffered boils – the reaction, they thought, to the drugs I was taking.

'The common perception is that arthritis is a disease for older people and that's certainly what I thought,' Stephen says. 'I just couldn't get my head around what the rheumatologists were saying, and I could not accept that I had arthritis.'

In 1993, he came out of hospital and started taking three drugs: Feldene, Salazopyrin and Naproxen. This, in itself, wasn't easy for Stephen who had always been anti-medication, loathed taking any tablets and prided himself on his fitness.

'The best way to describe what happened next,' says Stephen 'is that I had three years of turmoil. I wasn't able to continue my work as a financial adviser with an investment company, and I was getting flare-ups about every month. But between those times, it didn't seem right that I had arthritis, as I looked perfectly fit and healthy. At times I wanted to be carrying a label saying exactly what I had, just to prove it.'

For the first year of his illness, Stephen and his wife had to move in with his wife's mother, to help them to cope. 'My life was like a jigsaw puzzle thrown into the air – all the pieces scattered and no two things fitted together' he remembers.

Stephen had been in touch with Arthritis Care, to try to find out more about his condition, and they had sent him some literature. So strong was his sense of denial that he had completely ignored it at first, and binned the leaflets. But then Arthritis Care got in touch with him again and badgered him to go on an Arthritis Care course.

'Thank goodness I did, because until then, no one seemed to want to treat the emotional side of my illness. On the course, I met a trainer who listened and really wanted to know about my past, my sporting history and how I was feeling about not being able to continue that. He challenged everything that I believed about myself, the way that I was looking at my arthritis and the way that I was managing it. I wasn't looking after my diet, or my sleep patterns, and I was slipping into a disability mind-set.'

It was only then that Stephen started to accept that arthritis was part of him. 'Up until that point' he says 'I can honestly say that every morning I woke up and expected my arthritis to have gone.' This was the real turning-point for Stephen. Until then he felt that he and arthritis were two different things. 'The hardest part was accepting that arthritis was part of me' he remembers. 'Instead of fighting it, I had to embrace it; I now know that I am still the same person, but if I have to rest, then I lie down, and that's that. Once that was clear to me, things improved enormously.'

Now that he felt that he could move forward with this acceptance, he wanted to know more about arthritis and the

> **'I wasn't looking after my diet or sleep patterns, and I was slipping into a disability mind-set.'**

continued on page 60

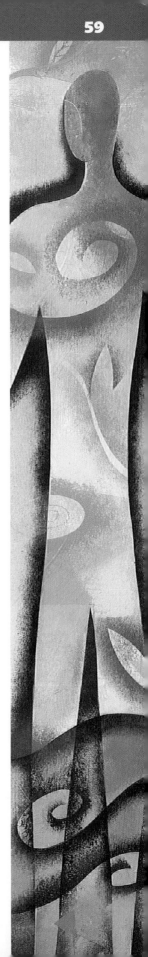

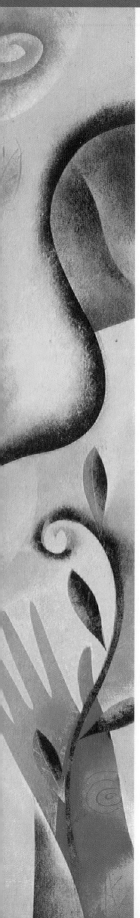

disability it can mean. Part of this meant he started a new way of eating, which at first struck him as very odd. 'But it seemed to work' he confirms. 'I started to stay off wheat – I stopped eating bread completely – no dairy products, pork, or anything with acidity in it. I love sandwiches, so it was hard to avoid bread, but I've kept it going to this day. I drink rice-milk wherever possible, and I can't eat wheat-based cereals, so I eat oat porridge. In fact, rice, broccoli, carrots, fish and chicken became my staple diet. I try to eat a lot of oily fish, like salmon and mackerel.'

The change in his diet ran alongside a lot of what Stephen learned through his AC trainer, such as relaxation, meditation and visualization. Visualization is a technique in which you visualize a situation and experience the positive and negative aspects of it. For instance, Stephen wanted to get fitter, but found the idea of visiting a leisure centre very daunting, knowing he had once been one of the best. 'So, to overcome this anxiety, I would visualize myself walking into a

> **'There are times when I wake up sore and stiff, but I haven't had a major flare-up for two years.'**

leisure centre and experiencing both the good and the difficult aspects of the situation. When it came to actually doing it, it was far less daunting, as I had already tried to cope with the specific anxieties I might face.'

He became involved with the work of Arthritis Care and, at the age of 34, went to the University of Ulster for a year, to follow a Diploma in Disability Studies.

'I was also asked to work as a mentor for personal development courses for those with a disability. I enjoyed that enormously, and it led me to make the link between coaching and my past sporting life.' To make coaching his career, Stephen knew he would need some form of qualification. Unfortunately, the MA course that he wanted to take was far too expensive, so he had to forget the idea.

However, he still had his good reputation as an athlete, and was asked to take a look at a promising new athlete from the point of view of a coach. He agreed, but says 'It was actually a horrible feeling – like waiting for your first driving lesson. I'd put on weight, I was going into an environment where everyone was fit and healthy and I was perhaps two and a half stone heavier than I was when I was competing. I began to regret agreeing to go along, and when the time came, it was like facing all my demons again.'

After visiting the athletics track, Stephen started coaching the athlete, and within a year she'd won an Irish senior long-jump title. Stephen was really making a difference, and people saw this. His coaching skills were being recognized on a national basis, and he was asked to become the national jumps coach for Ireland.

Stephen asks his athletes to visualize going out onto a big track and encountering strong competitors. 'This helps them hugely in preparing for a major event. It helps to combat nerves, increases confidence and can greatly improve technique. It works especially well for those who have been injured. I'm a great believer in the power of the mind' he says.

'Years ago, if someone had told me I was going to get arthritis, I would have laughed at them. But it happened. There was nothing I could do to stop that, and there have been a lot of tears, kicking and cursing. Then, if anyone had told me that I would

be back in sport, coaching this time, I would never have believed it. And of course, to be coaching at a national level, would have been inconceivable.

'I'm actually looking forward to seeing what is going to come up next! My life has turned around so very much.'

Two years ago, Stephen found he could get a bursary for the course he wanted to follow, and he recently completed his MA.

He is now developing his own coaching business, working with people who need help getting back to work after illness, and he is a trustee for Arthritis Care, for whom he gives motivational talks.

'My arthritis is now very manageable, I have learned to meditate, which I do every day, and my diet has improved to agree more with my body's needs. I still have to take Naproxen, and there are times when I will wake up and be sore and stiff, but I haven't had a major flare-up for two years now. It's down to the quality of my life: I'm not stressed about arthritis, and of course, I have the support of my wife and family.'

Stephen's latest wish is for the record he set 23 years ago to be broken by the promising young athlete he is coaching.

'Now that really would be a turnaround' he says with a smile.

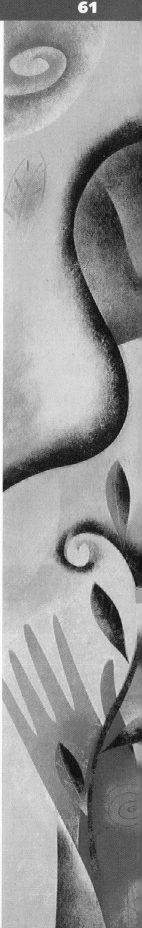

Type I diabetes, RA is an autoimmune disease, meaning that the body's immune system mistakenly attacks healthy tissue as if it were a foreign invader.

> ◘ **FACT** Rheumatoid arthritis can affect any of the body's freely movable joints, but most commonly involves the hands, wrists, shoulders, elbows, knees, ankles and feet.

RA's target This autoimmune attack is directed against the joint's synovial membrane. It inflames the joint and causes pain, warmth, stiffness and swelling – symptoms common to many types of arthritis. What distinguishes RA from all other forms of inflammatory arthritis is the potential for the inflamed synovial membrane to severely damage the joints. In addition, RA's inflammation may spread beyond the joints to affect other parts of the body. Fortunately, new disease-modifying drugs can block this destructive inflammation by deactivating the immune system components that attack the body's own tissues.

Researchers have identified risk factors that make some people more likely to develop RA than others. Chief among these risk factors is a person's genetic makeup.

The role of heredity

People who develop RA do seem to have inherited a susceptibility to the disease. Several different genes probably determine whether someone will have a tendency to develop RA and how severe his or her disease will be. As you might expect, these tend to be genes that control immune system function.

For example, some 65 per cent of people with RA have a genetic marker – a protein called HLA-DR4 – on the surface of their white blood cells. White cells play major roles in the body's effort to fight infections, so this protein may somehow 'mislead' white cells into attacking the body's own tissues.

A missing link Patients who have this genetic marker usually have more severe rheumatoid arthritis than those patients without it. However, fully one in four people who have the marker never develops rheumatoid arthritis, which shows that having 'RA genes' isn't sufficient to bring on the condition. Instead, researchers believe something must be present to trigger RA in susceptible people.

did you
know

◘ Almost 90 per cent of the joints that are ultimately affected in RA will be affected during the first year of the disease. So if you've had RA for several years, there is the consolation of knowing that the disease probably won't spread any further.

The search for a trigger. For nearly a century, researchers have looked for a link between dozens of infectious agents and the development of RA. Bacteria have long been prime suspects: since they were implicated in causing some types of arthritis, such as Reiter's syndrome, it made sense that bacteria could be involved in RA as well.

In 1912, an American rheumatologist proposed that RA occurred when bacterial toxins from localized infections in the tonsils, gums, teeth or gall bladder were carried to the joints via the bloodstream. This 'focal infection' theory failed to hold water, but for the next 30 years, unfortunate RA patients had their tonsils removed or all their teeth extracted in a vain effort to halt the progress of the disease.

To see if RA was contagious, researchers in 1950 took fluid from the joints of people with RA and injected it into the joints of healthy volunteers. None of the volunteers developed RA, providing conclusive evidence that RA does not involve a persistent infection of the joints.

In recent years, viruses have received the most attention as possible culprits in triggering RA. A prime suspect for more than a decade has been the Epstein-Barr virus, which causes mononucleosis. Studies show that susceptible people – those with any one of three genes associated with RA – tend to have an abnormal immune response to Epstein-Barr infections that may trigger RA.

Many arthritis experts remain convinced that infections can initiate RA. So far, the strenuous efforts to link a bacterium, virus or some other infectious agent to the condition have all failed. But even if some microbe eventually is implicated in causing RA, one thing seems certain: you can't 'catch' RA from someone else.

The oestrogen factor

Women are much more susceptible to autoimmune diseases than men, and RA is no exception: three out of every four people who develop RA are women, and researchers suspect the hormone oestrogen. Combined with certain 'susceptibility genes', oestrogen seems to tip the balance towards developing RA: For example, a woman who inherits the genes will very likely develop the disease, while a brother with the same genes will remain healthy. When a woman has a genetic tendency to develop RA,

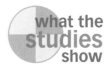

what the studies show

▶ A study published in 2000 supports the notion that Epstein-Barr infections could play a role in some cases of RA. Comparing 55 people with RA to people without, researchers from the University of Gottingen in Germany found that RA patients had double the levels of antibody against Epstein-Barr as people without RA. In addition, 14 of the RA patients had evidence of a reactivated Epstein-Barr infection compared with none of those without RA.

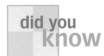

◗ Women with RA often find that their disease abates during pregnancy – sometimes remarkably so. Unfortunately, the disease usually resumes its severity a month or two after delivery. And in some women RA appears for the first time in the weeks following childbirth. Whatever causes 'pregnancy remissions' could help researchers to develop new treatments for RA.

now and
then

◗ Doctors once believed that damage to a joint's bones did not occur until many years after RA began affecting that joint. But recently, studies have shown that bone damage starts during the first year or two after RA's onset – pointing to the need for early diagnosis of RA and treatment to halt the inflammation that causes the damage.

oestrogen may supersensitize her immune system so that, in response to some infection, immune cells launch an attack on her tissues and the invading microbes.

How does RA progress?

In about 80 per cent of cases, RA begins slowly, affecting just a few joints at first, typically those in the fingers, wrists or toes. Eventually, the disease almost always ends up affecting 20 joints or more, including the shoulders, ankles, hips, knees and other joints. But not all cases develop gradually: RA sometimes appears seemingly overnight, involving many of the body's joints in just a matter of days.

If this inflammation of a joint's synovial membrane persists, the membrane's cells may begin growing uncontrollably, forming extra tissue called pannus and thickening the normally thin membrane. The joint becomes swollen and feels puffy to the touch.

A slow cascade of pain As RA progresses, the growing synovial membrane spreads and eventually covers the top of the joint cartilage. Invading cells from the thickened, inflamed synovial membrane release destructive enzymes that erode the cartilage and underlying bone of the joint and eventually weaken the muscles, tendons and ligaments that surround it.

In the later stages of RA, joints become so severely damaged that they can no longer function properly. The inflammation may totally erode the cartilage and deform a joint by causing bones to fuse together. Fortunately, the disease-modifying antirheumatic drugs available today, can prevent crippling and disability in many cases, if treatment begins early enough.

How is RA diagnosed?

RA can be notoriously difficult to diagnose, especially in its early stages. Usually, its symptoms don't appear all at once, but typically reveal themselves slowly, over months or years. Stiff, painful joints can be an early indication of RA, but they occur in many other joint diseases. For this reason, diagnosing RA often requires ruling out other possible causes of the symptoms.

Medical history

As with OA, the first step is for a doctor to take your medical history (see page 48). The answers to certain questions – 'Which joints are giving you trouble?', 'Do the joints feel stiff in

The four degrees of RA

No two cases of RA proceed in exactly the same way. In fact, experts stress that RA's course in any patient is quite unpredictable. But they have identified four basic ways in which the disease progresses – or, in some cases, doesn't.

1 In a few people – perhaps around 10 per cent who develop it – RA is a temporary problem: these people experience a spontaneous and lasting remission that can't be attributed to any treatment they might be undergoing. When they happen, these spontaneous remissions usually occur within the first two years that people have RA. Another 10 per cent of RA patients experience remissions, but the disease recurs later.

2 In the second type of RA, patients experience periodic flare-ups – weeks or months of painful, stiff and swollen joints – that alternate with intervals of normal health. Their treatment will depend on whether their joints are damaged during the flare-ups and how well their joints function between flare-ups.

3 In the third type of RA, known as remitting-progressive, patients experience periodic flare-ups without returning to normal health between the attacks. Instead, during the periods between attacks, they have lingering joint inflammation that becomes increasingly more severe with each attack. If it isn't treated properly, remitting-progressive RA can eventually lead to significant joint damage.

4 The fourth type is called progressive RA, which is self-explanatory: the inflammation becomes more severe over time and causes gradually increasing pain, swelling and – if severe inflammation lasts long enough – joint damage and disability.

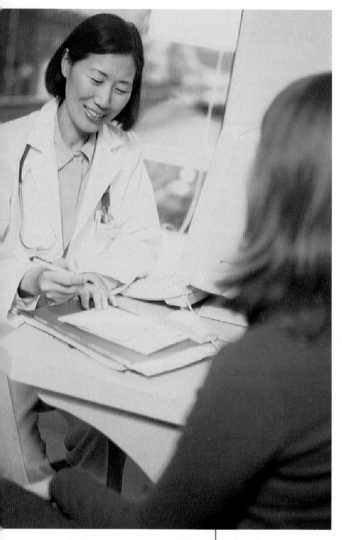

the morning and, if so, how long does the stiffness last?', 'Are you experiencing a lot of fatigue?' – can help a doctor to narrow down the list of possible joint problems.

Physical examination

The doctor will focus on the affected joints, looking for the tell-tale signs of RA: joints that are tender, reddened, swollen or warm, and have a limited range of motion. As noted earlier, problems in symmetrical joints, both elbows, for example, increase the odds that RA is present.

Laboratory test

Only one laboratory test is useful for confirming a diagnosis of RA; it is known as the rheumatoid factor test. Rheumatoid factor is an antibody produced by the synovial membranes of joints affected by RA and can be found in the blood of 80-90 per cent of people who have the condition. (Unfortunately, rheumatoid factor is often absent in the early stages of RA – when the test's help in diagnosing the disease is, in fact, most needed.) Generally, patients who test positive for rheumatoid factor tend to have more severe RA, and people with high levels of rheumatoid factor are more acutely affected than those with low amounts.

Blood cell test Another test, the erythrocyte sedimentation rate, or 'ESR', is a broad indicator of inflammation in the body, including rheumatoid arthritis. Inflammation tends to make red blood cells sticky, so they form clumps that will settle (form a sediment) in a test tube. The greater the inflammation, the larger the red-cell clumps and the faster they'll fall to the bottom of the tube. This makes the ESR a useful tool for monitoring whether a treatment for rheumatoid arthrits is reducing inflammation. But because infections, malignancies and other medical problems can provoke inflammation, the ESR is of limited help in diagnosing the condition.

Rheumatic rundown

Painful, swollen joints occur in a large number of joint ailments. Here is a list of rheumatic diseases with similar symptoms:

- Rheumatoid arthritis
- Ankylosing spondylitis
- Systemic lupus erythematosus
- Arthritis associated with psoriasis
- Reiter's syndrome
- Gout
- Pseudogout
- Bursitis

Fluid examination A useful but more invasive way to confirm that a person has some form of inflammatory arthritis is to evaluate synovial fluid removed from an affected joint by use of a needle. The fluid is examined under a microscrope to see if there are large numbers of neutrophils, white blood cells that gather at sites of inflammation.

X-rays

These are of limited use in diagnosing RA. They often appear totally normal early in the course of the disease, even when symptoms are severe. In fact, X-rays usually don't provide evidence of RA until significant and irreversible joint damage has occurred. At that point, X-rays reveal that inflammation has destroyed cartilage and eroded the underlying bone.

What now?

A diagnosis of RA can be sobering: the disease can cause significant joint damage and disability. It can disrupt people's lives, affecting their relationships and draining their financial resources. But you can blunt RA's impact if you approach the disease in the right way.

Don't panic The great majority of people who are diagnosed with RA have relatively mild symptoms that can be controlled with proper treatment. Furthermore, breakthrough treatments for RA have been introduced in just the past few years, and even better treatments are expected in the near future.

what the studies show

- In a large-scale study published in 1994, an average of nine months elapsed between the time RA patients first experienced symptoms and when they were finally diagnosed with RA.

Surviving flare-ups

For people diagnosed with any type of arthritis, 'flare-up' becomes an important part of their vocabulary. Things may be going along smoothly – so smoothly you've almost forgotten you have arthritis – and then, suddenly, a flare-up.

Arthritis flare-ups are times when things go wrong: inflammation, pain and stiffness resurface with a vengeance. They can be set off by many different things: overdoing things at the gym, lack of sleep, emotional stress.

Flare-ups can severely challenge the patience – sometimes even the sanity – of people with arthritis. Successfully taking charge of arthritis means riding out a flare-up so that it causes the least amount of aggravation and despair.

Minimizing pain The key is learning how to adjust to without giving in. When a flare-up occurs, you should give yourself more rest and protect the inflamed joints from further exertion. However, overprotecting a joint can be counterproductive, since long periods of inactivity can cause the muscles and tendons around a joint to weaken. You may also want to consult your doctor about adjusting your medication in response to a flare-up.

Unfortunately, these periodic crises are an unavoidable part of arthritis. But knowing that you can manage them means that you don't have to live in dread of them.

Tell your friends and family Even people with mild cases of RA can expect to experience periodic 'flares', which are sudden worsenings of the inflammation that can temporarily disable a person with pain and fatigue. If family and friends are aware of this and other RA complications, they'll be more understanding and willing to pitch in to help when you're not feeling up to par.

Getting the right care If you've been diagnosed with RA by your GP, he or she may then refer you to a rheumatologist – a senior doctor who specializes in diagnosing and treating all forms of arthritis. More than most other diseases, RA demands close monitoring and fine-tuning of treatment to prevent permanent damage to joints. As mentioned, all GPs should be familiar with treating RA and should know the latest treatments. As it is so important to have a good rapport with your doctor, you should have a GP or rheumatologist with whom you feel comfortable. If you don't, then get a second opinion.

Assemble a healthcare team Although it is unlikely that your GP will be the only person responsible for your treatment, he or she may be involved in monitoring it, and should be in close touch with the rest of the team. GPs can also put you in direct contact with a physiotherapist (who can help you to set up an exercise programmme), an occupational therapist (who can help you to cope with day-to-day tasks) and other professionals, such as dietitians. This help can also come through the hospital rheumatology unit.

Set realistic goals This is important for people with any type of arthritis but especially RA, a disease that can pose significant physical and emotional challenges. Setting and meeting realistic goals is vital to coping with the condition, and you can learn how to do that in this book.

Make use of resources. People with RA can benefit greatly from a wide variety of resources, including support groups and self-help courses sponsored by Arthritis Care and local support groups, and health information offered on the Internet.

How is RA treated?
In RA, patient and doctor work together to achieve several goals:

- ◉ alleviate pain, stiffness, swelling, fatigue and other symptoms

- ◉ reduce the inflammation

- ◉ slow down or halt the joint damage

- ◉ limit RA's interference with a patient's life

Drugs can put out the fire
Virtually all people diagnosed with RA must rely on drugs to control their disease. The arsenal of drugs used to treat it generally falls into two classes: NSAIDs (nonsteroidal

now and then

◉ Until the late 1980s, doctors believed that early RA could be managed exclusively with NSAIDs, and that disease-modifying antirheumatic drugs (DMARDs) weren't needed until joint damage showed up on X-rays. They later realized that permanent joint damage can occur even in the first months of RA – despite the use of NSAIDs and long before damage can be seen on X-rays. Now, experts agree that use of DMARDs should begin in the early stages after RA is diagnosed.

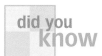

did you know

◉ Recent studies suggest that fewer people are developing rheumatoid arthritis than in previous years. A reduction in smoking and the use of oral contraceptives may be the reason.

Filtering out RA

In the United States, in March 1999, the FDA approved the Prosorba column, the first 'nondrug alternative' for adults with moderate to severe RA who cannot tolerate DMARDs. During a 2 hour process, the patient's blood is removed and passed through a machine that separates the plasma from the blood cells. The plasma is then passed through the Prosorba column, a device about the size of a coffee mug. The filtered plasma is then recombined with its blood cells, and the blood is reinfused into the patient.

The Prosorba treatment can cause dramatic improvement in RA patients. Although researchers don't fully understand the column's mechanism, they believe it filters out proteins involved in the immune system's attack on the joints. This treatment is not yet available in the UK.

anti-inflammatory drugs) and DMARDs (disease-modifying anti-rheumatic drugs). Successful treatment of RA, usually requires taking both types of drugs.

NSAIDs for inflammation NSAIDs are the mainstays of RA treatment. As their name implies, they reduce inflammation and the symptoms it causes, including pain, stiffness and swelling. NSAIDs include ordinary aspirin and other drugs such as diclofenac, ibuprofen, ketoprofen, naproxen, piroxicam, and sulindac. However, the high doses used in treating RA can cause a nasty side effect: serious gastrointestinal bleeding.

The first three of a new class of NSAIDs called COX-2 inhibitors have been licensed in the UK. These drugs, Celebrex, Vioxx and Mobic, relieve inflammation as well as standard NSAIDs, with less risk of causing gastrointestinal problems. These COX-2 inhibitors are useful for people over 65, who are especially susceptible to bleeding from using standard NSAIDs.

Although NSAIDs act against inflammation, they don't prevent renegade synovial tissue from eroding cartilage and bone – the destructive process that inflammation sets in motion, and that causes permanent joint damage.

DMARDs for joint damage Disease-modifying anti-rheumatic drugs (DMARDs) resemble NSAIDs in that they help to dampen RA's inflammation. But more importantly, the DMARDs can alter the course of RA by slowing down or halting the joint damage that can occur independently of inflammation.

DMARDs are slow-acting drugs, and it may take several weeks before their effects are noticeable. People taking DMARDs must be closely monitored, because these drugs have the potential for causing serious adverse side effects.

For nearly 20 years, methotrexate – a drug first approved as a cancer treatment – has been the most widely prescribed DMARD. But three new DMARDs approved in the United States since 1998 have greatly enhanced the treatment of RA and have already transformed the lives of many people with the disease.

The next generation Two of these new DMARDs – Enbrel (etanercept) and Remicade (infliximab) – are drugs that are genetically engineered to neutralize tumour necrosis factor, a chemical that seems to play a major role in causing both inflammation and joint damage.

Arava (leflunomide) is the third new DMARD and the only one that can be taken orally (all other DMARDs must be injected). Arava retards RA's progression by blocking an enzyme in white blood cells involved in the immune system's attack on the joints.

caution

Rheumatoid arthritis is often swiftly treated with powerful drugs, which can have serious side effects. Be patient. If the diagnosis is unclear, have the condition assessed over weeks or months: a 'true' case will reveal itself in time.

Surgery for better mobility

When RA's joint damage is severe, several types of surgical repair are possible. Total joint replacement with an artificial joint can dramatically reduce pain and improve function in RA patients.

Excellent results are now achieved in the replacement of knees, hips and shoulders, but the outcome is less certain when elbows, wrists, and ankles are replaced.

Fibromyalgia – the pain is real

If you literally ache all over, you may have fibromyalgia (FM) – one of the most distressing of all medical problems. One recent textbook described FM as a 'chronic, poorly understood and disabling condition'. It is all of that and more.

FM is relatively common, affecting more than a million Britons, or 2 per cent of the general population. The overwhelming majority of FM patients – more than 90 per cent – are women, and the ailment typically starts when a person is in her mid 40s. Fibromyalgia is a significant health problem, accounting for 20 per cent of visits that people make to rheumatologists.

What is FM?

FM's main features are severe and widespread muscle pain that is most pronounced in the neck and shoulders, extreme fatigue, and – in most cases – poor sleep. Fibromyalgia can feel like a joint disease, but the pain actually occurs in nearby muscles, ligaments, and tendons.

FM's pain and other symptoms may persist for years – even for life – but may vary in intensity from day to day. Both inactivity and unaccustomed physical activity can make symptoms worse, as can insomnia, humid weather and stress.

In addition to widespread persistent pain, fatigue and poor sleep, people with FM typically report many other problems including:

did you know

◗ Patients with fibromyalgia often have symptoms of spastic colon, which include abdominal pain, alternating diarrhoea and constipation, gas and bloating. Peppermint oil can be helpful. Although it eases spasms in the colon, it can cause indigestion in the stomach, so it is important to use enteric-coated peppermint oil capsules that are made not to dissolve until they pass the stomach.

- Irritable bowel syndrome (in up to 50 per cent of cases)

- Tension headache

- Problems concentrating or remembering

- Sense of swollen hands that are normal on examination

- Palpitations

- Depression

What causes FM?

One of the most frustrating aspects of FM – for patients, their families, and their doctors – is the absence of any definite cause or causes. FM may well be the result of a complex interaction of many different physiological and psychological factors. Experts have proposed a number of theories for what causes FM, including:

Heredity or family history

Research shows that FM patients are more likely to have a family history of pain, depression or alcoholism than other people. Also, not surprisingly, FM is more common among relatives of FM patients than among relatives of nonaffected people.

The stress factor

Most researchers agree that stress is a key factor in FM. Studies show that FM patients report high levels of stress in their lives – more, for example, than in rheumatoid arthritis patients or in other people who don't have FM.

A recent study involving FM patients found that the greater their psychological distress, the more sensitive they are to pain and the more physical complaints they have. What's not clear is whether stress causes FM or is the consequence of living with a severe and sometimes disabling condition.

A real problem Even if stress does cause FM, the disorder clearly isn't 'all in the mind', as some sceptics contend, but is a genuine medical problem. Mind-body research over the past decade shows that emotional stress can cause major changes in the body that adversely affect the nervous system and immune system, as well as hormone levels.

now and then

- Until about 20 years ago FM was known as fibrositis, a condition of inflamed muscles, tendons and other fibrous tissues. In 1979, Canadian physicians showed that fibrositis patients also suffered from extreme fatigue and, in almost all cases, had problems with sleep. Studies also found that the aching joints of fibrositis patients were not actually inflamed. So in 1981 Dr. Muhammad B. Yunus, professor of medicine at the University of Illinois College of Medicine at Peoria, proposed the term 'fibromyalgia', which roughly means aching muscles and other soft tissues. In the UK, FM was formally recognized as a medical disorder in 1992, when the Arthritis Research Campaign put together a set of criteria.

High levels of substance P

Substance P, which is a chemical responsible for alerting the nervous system to a painful injury of the tissues, is found at elevated levels in the cerebrospinal fluid of people with fibromyalgia. In some people with FM, levels of substance P consistently measure two to three times above normal; in others, the levels gradually increase as symptoms become more severe. Increased substance P levels, perhaps induced by stress, may help to explain the recent finding that FM patients have a lower pain threshold (greater sensitivity to pain) than people who don't have the condition.

Injuries, accidents or traumas

Some people can trace the onset of their FM to relatively minor accidents such as bumper-bashing collisions. But most experts doubt that minor trauma can produce the long-lasting effects on muscles and other soft tissue throughout the body that characterizes FM.

Tendering a diagnosis of FM

The 18 tender points are nine paired points (the insides of both elbows, for example) on the front and back of the body between the knees and the neck (see above). Pressing the tender points firmly will hurt anyone; but in someone with FM, pressing tender points lightly, with just enough pressure to cause the fingernail to blanch, can cause excruciating pain.

A diagnosis of fibromyalgia requires pain in at least 11 of these tender points. But as a practical matter, experts believe that someone with long-standing musculoskeletal pain, plus impaired sleep that doesn't relieve fatigue, can still be diagnosed with FM even if fewer than 11 tender points are painful to the touch.

Taking charge of fibromyalgia

Sometimes it's easier to have a clear-cut medical problem than one like FM, with its largely subjective symptoms of pain and fatigue. People with FM must often contend with sceptical doctors and family members who doubt whether their complaints are real.

Hands-on benefits For this and other reasons, including a lack of truly effective treatments, FM can be an especially difficult illness to cope with, but also one that can be greatly helped by the take-charge approach of this book. Studies consistently show that by gaining self-empowerment – believing in your ability to control your disease and overcome symptoms – FM patients can improve their mood, decrease pain and better tolerate the pain they still have.

How is FM diagnosed?

A striking feature of FM is that standard diagnostic tests – blood tests or X-rays, for example – appear perfectly normal. As a result, a diagnosis of FM must be made by clinical examination.

In 1990, after comparing FM patients with control patients, the American College of Rheumatology set out specific criteria for doctors to use in diagnosing FM. These criteria are also widely accepted in the UK. To be diagnosed with FM, patients must be experiencing:

◐ Widespread muscle pain that has been present for at least three months

◐ Pain in at least 11 of 18 'tender points' when a doctor presses on those spots

◐ **FACT** Fibromyalgia is the most frequently seen musculoskeletal disorder in UK rheumatology clinics.

What now?

If you're like many people, you may actually be relieved to receive a diagnosis of FM: some people spend years seeking an explanation for their symptoms, with numerous doctors telling them that the problem is all in their head.

Accentuate the positive The good news for people with fibromyalgia is that it doesn't involve damage to the joints. Even though you may hurt all over and feel exhausted, you won't be crippled by FM. On the other hand, FM tends to linger, sometimes for life, although the severity of the pain and fatigue may ebb and flow over the years. One of the keys to coping with FM is overcoming the sleep disturbances that contribute to FM's sometimes disabling fatigue.

How is FM treated?

Since there is no known cause for FM, treatment is aimed at easing its symptoms – not an easy task. For example, drugs that work well at relieving pain associated with many types of arthritic problems (ibuprofen and other NSAIDs) are notably ineffective against the pain of fibromyalgia. This difficulty in

Fibromyalgia strategy guide: what else you can do

- Eat several small meals during the day to maintain a steady supply of protein and carbohydrate for proper muscle function.
- Take hot baths or showers – especially in the morning – to soothe soreness, increase circulation and relieve stiffness.
- Find a massage therapist familiar with fibromyalgia. A technique called trigger-point therapy can be extremely helpful in reducing pain.
- Cut back on caffeine, alcohol and sugar, which often cause fatigue.
- Try to get at least 8 hours of sleep a night – aerobics or certain antidepressants may improve sleep quality.

finding effective treatments often only adds to the frustration that many fibromyalgia patients may experience.

Exercise Although no one treatment has proven universally effective against FM, doctors who have cared for many FM patients seem to agree that aerobic exercise should be a part of any treatment programme. Aerobic exercise improves sleep – almost always poor among FM patients – and better sleep helps relieve FM's extreme fatigue. In addition, studies also show that aerobic exercise helps to ease muscle pain and tenderness in FM patients.

Many fibromyalgia patients find that the best route to the relief of their symptoms is a combination of different treatments. Some US studies, for instance, have suggested that combinations of magnesium and malic acid, L-carnitine and co-enzyme Q-10, when taken with a high-potency multivitamin/antioxidant combination, may help FM patients. Other possible treatments for FM include:

Low doses of antidepressants These drugs – tricyclics like amitriptyline and SSRIs like Prozac – are given mainly to improve sleep and relax muscles rather than to relieve depression. Both types of drug seem to have physiological effects on the nervous system that may explain the improvement in fatigue and nonrejuvenating sleep experienced by people with FM. In general, drugs that improve sleep have proven to be the most useful medications for treating fibromyalgia.

NSAIDs These painkilling drugs have generally proven disappointing in clinical studies involving FM patients. But some people with FM may benefit from using them.

Topical treatments Applying creams containing capsaicin, a substance derived from chilli peppers, to painful areas seems to help some FM sufferers because capsaicin reduces levels of substance P in sensitive nerve endings; the levels of the substance are often increased in fibromyalgia patients and have been linked to their lower pain threshold. But this beneficial effect can take two or three weeks. Meanwhile the patient may suffer temporary side effects of skin-reddening and irritation.

Acupuncture This ancient treatment has shown promise in treating several types of musculoskeletal problems, including FM.

caution

FM patients embarking on an exercise programme should start out slowly, especially if they've been inactive, since unaccustomed exertion can cause severe pain. You should also avoid high-impact exercises – jogging or tennis, for example – and opt for cycling, walking or swimming instead.

what the studies show

In one study, published in 1992 in the *British Medical Journal*, 70 FM patients were randomly assigned to receive six treatments using either electro-acupuncture (electric current is applied to the needles) or superficial 'needling'. At the end of the treatment period, patients receiving genuine acupuncture treatment were experiencing significantly less pain than patients receiving the sham treatment.

Ankylosing spondylitis: back pain with a twist

In the UK today there are 100,000 people clinically diagnosed with AS, a chronic inflammation of the spine. It is almost three times more common in men than in women, but it is possible that the ratio may be much more equal: women often have much milder cases that usually escape detection.

AS is mainly a disease of young people, and most commonly affects those between 15 and 35. Once thought to be part of rheumatoid arthritis, we now know that it is related but separate.

What is AS?

AS is a type of chronic arthritis that mainly affects the spine. (*Ankylosing* means stiff, *spondyl* refers to the spine, and *itis* means inflammation.) In AS, the inflammation occurs in joints and in areas where tendons and ligaments attach to bones. In severe cases, inflammation of the spine can actually cause the spinal vertebrae to fuse.

Older people who walk hunched over and looking down at the ground are usually in the late stages of AS. The good news is that today's treatments can almost always prevent AS from becoming a disabling or crippling condition.

What causes AS?

As with many types of arthritis, the cause of AS is not known. But genes have a strong influence, since 95 per cent of people who suffer from AS in the UK, have a genetic cell marker, or protein, called HLA-B27 on the surface of white blood cells. Someone who carries the HLA-B27 gene has a 1-2 per cent risk of developing AS, but the risk can rise to 20 per cent if a parent or sibling has the disease.

How does AS progress?

AS typically begins gradually, almost insidiously. The first symptoms are usually aches and pains in the lower back caused by inflammation of the sacroiliac joints, located in the lower back on both sides of the spine and just above the buttocks.

(Lower back pain that begins gradually and persists for months is often a tip-off for the disease.) The backache can be quite severe, interfering with sleep and causing a person to roll sideways to avoid bending the back when getting out of bed.

> **● FACT** One way to distinguish between a ruptured disc and early ankylosing spondylitis is that while disc pain is improved with rest, the pain of AS usually gets worse with rest and better with movement.

Ascending pain As it progresses, AS and its inflammation may move to the upper back and spread to other joints, especially the neck, hips and shoulders. The spine becomes stiff due to pain and muscle spasms. In the final stages, chronic inflammation can cause bony bridges to form between the vertebrae, resulting in the spine fusing permanently into a bent and inflexible position.

AS is a systemic disease, so it sometimes affects areas of the body beyond the joints. People with AS may experience fatigue, weight loss, poor appetite and – in about 25 per cent of patients – an inflammatory eye condition known as iritis, which causes redness and tearing. People with severe and long-standing AS may experience damage to heart tissue that requires the implantation of a pacemaker.

How is AS diagnosed?
Ankylosing spondylitis can be a challenging disease to diagnose, especially in its early stages. In general, the medical history alone can offer a doctor several clues that, when pieced together, point to a diagnosis of AS:

● The patient is a male between 16 and 35.

● Back pain and stiffness developed gradually.

● Symptoms have been present continually for more than three months.

● The patient has back stiffness on waking up in the morning.

● Exercise helps to relieve the stiffness and pain.

did you know

● Ankylosing spondylitis can be traced back to antiquity. In 1912, archaeologists unearthed an Egyptian mummy from about 3000 BC. The mummy's spine was described as 'a rigid block of stone' extending from its base to the neck.

The physical examination

The doctor will assess the flexibility of a patient's spine, asking him to bend over to touch his toes, for example. The doctor may also press on the patient's sacroiliac joints to see if they are tender and measure his lung function to see if the patient has trouble inhaling completely.

Laboratory tests

Testing the patient's blood for the presence of the HLA-B27 marker can help to confirm a diagnosis of AS or help to rule out similar diseases such as rheumatoid arthritis or lupus. Otherwise, diagnostic tests are not very useful in AS.

X-rays

These can provide a definitive diagnosis of AS, but signs of the disease usually don't show up on an X-ray until about five years after the disease begins. The first joints to show signs of ankylosing spondylitis are usually the sacroiliac joints, which appear fuzzy on X-rays because their surfaces have been eroded by inflammation.

> ⊙ **FACT** Tenderness where a tendon attaches to a bone – a sharp pain in the shoulders, buttocks, back of the knees or the heel – can be a sign of early-stage ankylosing spondylitis.

what the studies show

⊙ In studies of people with AS, the disease levelled off in almost all of them, but as many as 40 per cent had restricted joint movement of the spine. Also, in the vast majority of AS sufferers, breathing ability was impaired.

What now?

Someone recently diagnosed with AS should feel reasonably hopeful. Chances are you've been diagnosed early in the course of the disease. Today's treatments – primarily exercise and the use of NSAIDs – can almost always prevent AS from progressing to the point of irreversible spinal rigidity. They also do a good job of alleviating pain and stiffness and enable most people with ankylosing spondylitis to remain active and lead normal lives.

How is AS treated?

Today's treatments allow most people with AS to lead normal lives, but a take-charge approach emphasizing exercise is absolutely essential for success.

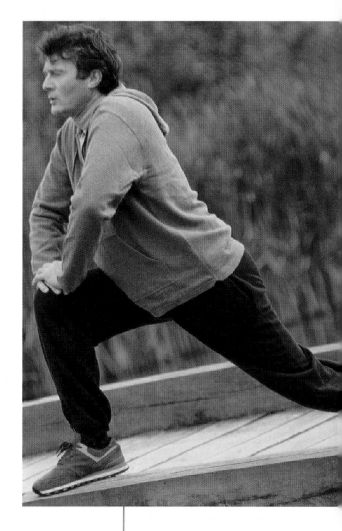

The healing power of exercise The outcome of AS can be greatly influenced by physiotherapy. A physiotherapist will teach you an exercise routine for daily use, and remind you to be aware of your posture. You will also learn how to increase the range of movement of certain joints, particularly your shoulders and hips. You also need to learn how to stretch the muscles that have become shortened. The National Ankylosing Spondylitis Society runs supervised weekly group physiotherapy sessions, through their local branches.

Although osteopathy and chiropractic are useful for some conditions, they are not recommended for sufferers of AS, because the manipulation can be inappropriate.

Drug therapy Regular use of NSAIDs is also important in treating AS – mainly because of its effect on exercise. These anti-inflammatory drugs ease pain and stiffness enough to allow patients to engage in an active exercise programme, which is critical in preventing the disease from worsening.

Systemic lupus erythematosus: the great impostor

Lupus is a chronic disease that usually inflames the joints, and also affects the skin, kidneys, blood vessels, nervous system and virtually every other organ in the body. About 1 in 750 women can be afflicted with lupus; women are about nine times more likely to have it than men. It is mainly a disease of young women, and in ethnic minority races, its occurrence is even greater: in Jamaica, one woman in 250 is affected.

did you know

Before corticosteroids were available, the mortality rate was high for lupus. Most people with serious kidney disease died and those without renal disease survived in only 50 per cent of cases.

People with lupus may want to avoid alfalfa in any form – including sprouts, seeds, tablets and tea. It contains a substance called canavanine, which some experts think can trigger flare-ups, although it is by no means a universal problem.

What is lupus?

Lupus is an autoimmune disease in which the immune system produces large numbers of several different types of antibody that attack the body's own tissues, causing symptoms that strongly resemble those of rheumatoid arthritis.

What causes lupus?

Experts believe people inherit a susceptibility to lupus: it is known to affect identical twins, and first-degree relatives of patients are much more likely than other people to develop the disease. In lupus, the body makes antibodies that attack the nuclei and other components of its own cells.

FACT Discoid lupus is limited to the skin. Symptoms include a rash on the face, neck and scalp. This type of lupus does not affect internal organs.

Some triggering event, such as an infection or stress, may provoke lupus in genetically susceptible people. Since lupus is almost always a disease that strikes young women, hormones may also play a role in causing it.

Drug-induced lupus Interestingly, many drugs commonly used to treat other diseases can cause temporary lupus, which disappears when the drug is stopped. Hydralazine (a high-blood-pressure medication), minocycline (used to treat acne) procainamide (used to treat irregular heartbeats) and isoniazid (a tuberculosis drug) are the chief culprits. This finding has attracted the attention of researchers who are studying how the drugs alter the immune system – findings that could shed light on how lupus develops and lead to better treatments.

How does lupus progress?

In the most typical cases, a young woman will develop an array of symptoms over several months that may include worsening fatigue, unexplained weight loss, a mild fever and a great deal of joint pain that doesn't involve swelling or joint tenderness. About half of people with early lupus will also develop a butterfly shaped facial rash that people once thought resembled a wolf's face – hence the name *lupus* (Latin for wolf). This distinctive rash can help in diagnosis.

Later in the course of the disease, other parts of the body may become affected, including the gastrointestinal tract (nausea, abdominal pain), blood cells (anaemia), tissue surrounding the heart and lungs (inflammation) and the nervous system (headaches, seizures, strokes and hallucinations). The kidneys are an especially important target, and damage to the organs can lead to kidney failure in late-stage lupus.

Other health problems that may occur in the later stages of lupus include cognitive problems such as decreased memory and difficulty doing simple mathematical calculations. In addition, sufferers are at risk of potentially fatal heart attack as a result of atherosclerosis.

How is lupus diagnosed?

Since it can affect so many parts of the body, lupus can mimic many diseases, making diagnosis very difficult, especially in the early stages of the condition. Presence of the butterfly rash can certainly help a doctor to make the diagnosis, but a definitive

'Sticky blood' may be the culprit

A major advance in the UK was the recognition in 1983 of 'sticky blood', the Antiphospholipid Syndrome (APS), sometimes known as Hughes' syndrome as it was first described by Dr. Graham Hughes, Head of the Lupus Research Unit at St Thomas' Hospital in London. It is now recognized as a significant part of the symptoms in some lupus patients.

Symptoms vary from headache, migraine, memory loss and fatigue, to clots in the vein and more serious problems. APS has become a big issue for doctors who realize that not all lupus manifestations require steroids – some require aspirin to thin blood in milder cases, and Warfarin where clotting has been a major problem. There are successes with many patients whose condition improved, once they started Warfarin treatment. Dr. Hughes says 'It has always been my belief that APS will one day come to be recognized as being more common than lupus.'

diagnosis sometimes depends on two tests that detect antibodies in the blood. These antibodies – antinuclear antibodies and anti-DNA antibodies – attack the nucleus of a patient's cells.

Lupus litmus tests Virtually all lupus patients test positive on the antinuclear antibody (ANA) test, which makes it a very good screening test for the condition. But people who have other types of arthritis, including rheumatoid arthritis, can also test positive. So patients who are suspected of having lupus, and who test positive on the ANA test, are given the anti-DNA antibody test, which is highly specific for the condition.

What now?

Lupus can certainly be a very serious disease. On the plus side, most people with lupus can be effectively treated. Especially over the past 30 years, treatment for lupus has dramatically improved, and some of the worst complications – such as kidney failure – can now almost always be avoided.

Lupus and fertility As most people diagnosed with lupus are young women, many are concerned that the condition may impair their ability to have children. Here again the news is largely reassuring: in women severely affected by lupus, the disease may indeed impair fertility and cause more frequent miscarriages. But the great majority of women with lupus can become pregnant and have healthy babies.

How is lupus treated?

Milder forms of lupus can usually be managed with nonsteroidal anti-inflammatory drugs such as apirin or ibuprofen, which reduce inflammation and pain. In more serious cases, when lupus affects the kidneys or other major organs, patients are usually given corticosteroids – potent anti-inflammatory drugs that can also cause serious side effects. Some two-thirds of lupus patients are treated with corticosteroids. In the most severe lupus cases, patients are treated with immunosuppressants – powerful drugs used to prevent a transplant recipient from rejecting a donated organ. They work in a similar way in lupus patients, by suppressing the immune system's attack on the body's organs.

Other types of arthritis: in a nutshell

Below and on the next four pages you will find only a small number of the types of arthritis you may be suffering from. Don't use these nutshell descriptions as a way of diagnosing your aches and pains. Make an appointment with your doctor and undergo a thorough physical examination. Your symptoms are unique and only your doctor can determine what you may have.

Finding the appropriate specialist is an important part of diagnosing your symptoms. It may take time to rule out the many other disorders that mimic your particular manifestation of arthritis before your doctor can make a final diagnosis. Once again, you and your doctor are partners in this important diagnosis process.

Reiter's syndrome: it starts with an infection

Reiter's syndrome is a chronic, intermittent, inflammatory condition that affects not only the joints (usually starting in the knees, feet or ankles) but also other parts of the body as well, particularly the urethra and the eyes, which can develop conjunctivitis. The syndrome is most common in men aged 20 to 40, who develop it after becoming infected with a sexually transmitted disease, and it also occurs in people with a genetic susceptibility traceable to the HLA-B27 gene.

> **FACT** Reiter's syndrome is called a reactive arthritis because the joint inflammation appears to be a reaction to an infection originating in an area other than the joints.

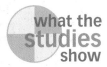

what the studies show

New studies show that microbes commonly cause rheumatoid arthritis and other rheumatic diseases in chimpanzees, rats, swine, poultry and other domestic animals. The two culprits are mycoplasmas and chlamydia – parasitic bacteria that produce Reiter's syndrome in the connective tissue of genetically susceptible people.

Causes and symptoms The condition is caused by the body's abnormal response to infections (either sexually transmitted diseases or infections of the gastrointestinal tract). Symptoms include inflammation of the urethra, conjunctivitis and joint pain and inflammation – usually of the knees and toes and areas where tendons are attached to bones, such as the heels.

The combination of joint, genital, urinary, skin and eye symptoms leads a doctor to suspect Reiter's syndrome. Because these symptoms may not appear simultaneously, the disease may not be diagnosed for several months. No simple laboratory tests are available to confirm the diagnosis.

What can be done Antibiotics are used to treat the infection and NSAIDs can minimize pain and inflammation in the joint. Although the patient often recovers, the arthritic symptoms may continue off and on for many years.

Gout: the arthritis of kings

Gout attacks occur when excess levels of uric acid in the blood form needle-like crystals that typically settle in one of the joints – most commonly in the big toe but sometimes in the knee or knuckles. Once in the joint, these abrasive particles can cause excruciating pain and inflammation. The condition has afflicted royalty and the well-to-do throughout the ages. However, it is by no means rare: it affects 16 men in every thousand, but only 3 women in every thousand – who rarely suffer from it before the menopause.

Causes and symptoms It's uncertain what precipitates a gout attack, though some factors may put you at risk. A quarter of those who suffer from gout have a family history of the illness, and three-quarters have high triglyceride levels.

Men who gain considerable weight between 20 and 40 are particularly vulnerable. Excessive alcohol intake, high blood pressure, kidney disease, exposure to lead, crash diets and certain medications (including antibiotics, diuretics and cancer chemotherapy drugs) may also play a role. For some people, eating foods high in chemicals called purines (such as liver or anchovies) can cause flare-ups.

Gout is diagnosed by identifying uric acid crystals in synovial fluid, usually by removing fluid from the joint through a needle. X-rays can be helpful and may reveal uric acid deposits and bone damage if you have suffered from repeated inflammations.

what the studies show

One study showed that eating fresh or canned cherries (8oz a day) may help to keep gout at bay by reducing levels of uric acid. Strawberries, blueberries, celery or celery seed extract may have a similar beneficial effect.

> ● **FACT** Drinking plenty of water, up to a litre or 2 pints a day, helps to increase the excretion of uric acid.

What can be done Avoiding purine-rich foods (liver and anchovies, seafoods, dried peas and beans) can help to prevent gout attacks.

Keeping your weight down can also help, as does avoiding foods that are high in fat and refined carbohydrates. Research studies have found that omega-3 fatty acids can decrease the body's output of inflammatory compounds. Gout-sufferers may find fish-oil supplements that contain omega-3 fatty acids can offer some relief for painful swelling of the joints.

The biggest treatment advance in managing gout is drugs such as allopurinol, probenecid (a drug given only by special arrangement) and sulfinpyrazone, that prevent gout attacks by controlling uric acid levels in the blood. The drug colchicine, derived from the autumn crocus, is one of the oldest known remedies for gout. But a newer, injectable form of the drug appears to work quickly and without side effects.

Pseudogout: a condition of the aged

This condition is very similar to gout but is caused by different types of crystal – in this case, calcium pryophosphate dihydrate crystals, which typically form for no reason. Pseudogout is common among older people, affecting about 3 per cent of people in their 60s and as many as half of all people over 90.

Causes and symptoms Although the cause of pseudogout is unknown, it may occur in people who have an abnormally high calcium level in the blood, an abnormally high iron level in the tissues or abnormally low blood levels of magnesium.

Symptoms of pseudogout vary widely. Some people have attacks of painful arthritis, usually in the knees, wrists, or other relatively large joints. Other people have lingering, chronic pain and stiffness in the joints of the arms and legs, which doctors may confuse with rheumatoid arthritis. Pseudogout is usually diagnosed in the same manner as gout – by removing fluid from the joint through a needle.

What can be done NSAIDs are used to reduce pain and inflammation and colchicine may be given intravenously to relieve the inflammation and pain during attacks.

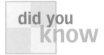
did you know

● According to the Arthritis Research Campaign (ARC), 250,000 people consult their GPs in the UK, every year, with a diagnosis of gout. The ratio of men to women is 3.8:1.

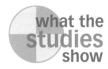

Polymyositis: attack of the muscles

Characterized by painful inflammation and degeneration of the muscles, polymyositis is a chronic connective tissue disease. It occurs in adults aged from 40 to 60 or in children from 5 to 15 years. Women are twice as likely as men to develop it.

Causes and symptoms Although the cause is unknown, viruses or auto-immune reactions may play a role. Cancer may also trigger the disease. Symptoms, which may begin during or just after an infection, include muscle weakness (particularly in the upper arms, hips and thighs), muscle and joint pain, a rash, difficulty in swallowing, a fever, fatigue and weight loss.

Polymyositis is often diagnosed by measuring muscle weakness at the shoulders or hips, or detecting a characteristic rash or increased blood levels of certain muscle enzymes.

What can be done Restricting your activities when the inflammation is most intense often helps. Generally, a cortico-steroid (usually prednisolone), taken orally, slowly increases strength and relieves pain and swelling, controlling the disease. In some cases, though, prednisolone actually worsens the disease. In these cases, immunosuppressive drugs are used instead of, or in addition to, prednisolone.

Psoriatic arthritis: from skin to joints

Although it resembles rheumatoid arthritis, psoriatic arthritis doesn't produce the antibodies characteristic of RA. A negative rheumatoid factor test helps to distinguish it from rheumatoid arthritis. It affects about 10 per cent of people who have the skin disease psoriasis. Psoriatic arthritis may develop at any age, but typically between the ages of 30 and 50, with heredity appearing to play a significant role in susceptibility.

Causes and symptoms Psoriasis (a skin condition causing flare-ups of red, scaly rashes and thickened, pitted nails) may precede or follow the joint inflammation. Psoriatic arthritis usually affects joints of the fingers and toes. The joints may become swollen and deformed when inflammation is chronic.

What can be done Treatment is aimed at controlling the rash and alleviating the joint inflammation. Several drugs that are effective in treating rheumatoid arthritis are also used to treat psoriatic arthritis. They include gold compounds, methotrexate, cyclosporin and sulfasalazine. Another drug, etretinate, is usually effective in severe cases, but its side effects may be serious.

Juvenile idiopathic arthritis: childhood pain

The catch-all name of juvenile idiopathic arthritis (JIA) is used to cover a number of types of arthritis. 'Idiopathic' means that doctors do not yet know its cause. In the UK, about 12,000 children suffer from JIA; the ratio of boys to girls is 1:2.5.

Causes and symptoms JIA can start at any age, and some forms may be difficult to detect. Oligoarticular JIA is by far the commonest and mildest form. It starts slowly, at the age of two or three, and affects fewer than four joints. Polyarthritis starts much earlier – in the first six months – and affects more than four joints. Systemic disease (or Still's disease) affects the whole body and causes not just inflamed joints, but high fever, rashes and other problems. There are other, rarer, types of arthritis, too.

Because it is so difficult to diagnose, especially in very young children, JIA can go undetected. Slowness to walk, or stopping walking a few months after starting, is one symptom. However, general moodiness, irritability and stiffness after sleep may all indicate tests should be taken.

What can be done Testing, such as MRI scans, may have to be done in hospital under an anaesthetic, as small children can find it hard to stay still for long. Depending on the type of arthritis your child has, treatment may involve drugs and a course of physiotherapy. In addition to scans and blood tests, your child's eyes will be tested. Eye tests are very important because children with arthritis are at risk of uveitis (inflammation of the eye), which, if left untreated, can cause blindness.

Because childhood arthritis can affect the whole family, a really consistent programme of exercises and activities should be worked out with your team of healthcare specialists, which will include your GP, a paediatrician, a rheumatologist (or an expert in both disciplines, known as a paediatric rheumatologist), an eye specialist and even a physiotherapist.

The key to the best care for your child is early treatment with effective medicines and an active exercise programme. Making sure your child has the best treatment, as soon as possible, will slow down the disease and reduce long-term damage to joints. Making exercise fun, and not a chore, will help to keep your child as mobile as possible.

Many children go into remission: the disease disappears for lengths of time – and, sometimes, forever – and very few fail to recover at all. Positive management is the key to containment.

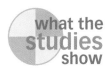

what the studies show

A 1997 study reported that gentle massage by parents for 15 minutes a day, can reduce a child's pain and stress.

did you know

Arthritis and some drug treatments can delay the onset of puberty for a few years in some children. This can cause self-consciousness in the child, and invoke teasing by other children. One of the advantages for the child, however, is that young people with disabilities on the Higher Rate Disability Living Allowance can get a provisional driving licence and drive a car at 16 – a year earlier than normal.

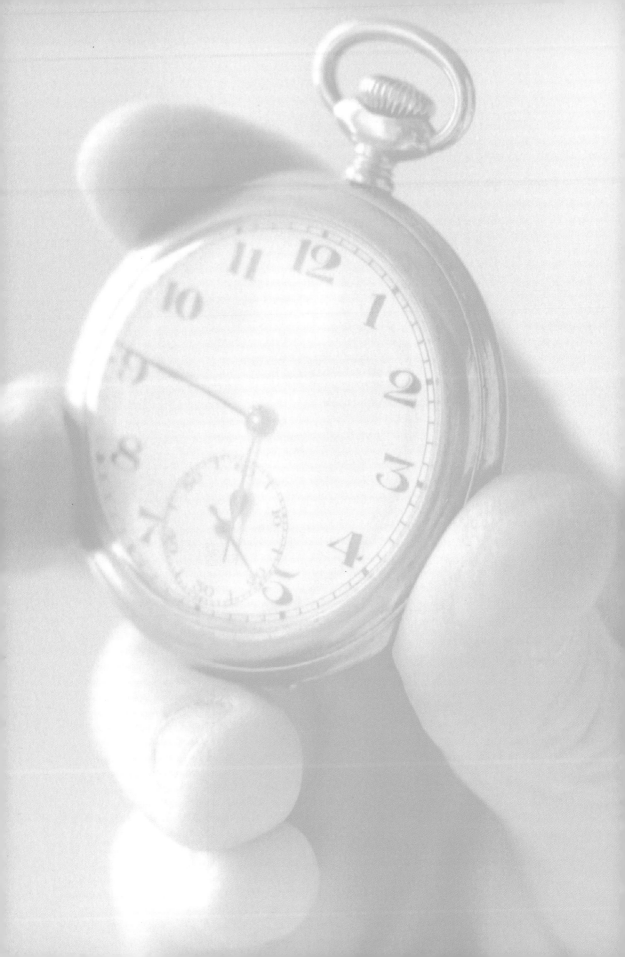

3

Taking charge now

As you take charge of your arthritis,

you will experience a sense of

self-empowerment. This will help you

not only to manage your condition

but also to avoid the depression

and feelings of hopelessness that

often afflict arthritis patients.

Chronic illness – what works for arthritis

Acute and chronic health problems are very different. Acute health problems appear abruptly and do not last long; typically, they either get better on their own or respond promptly to treatment.

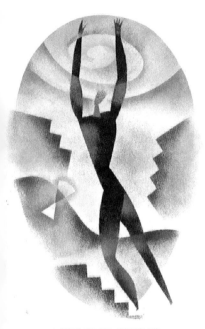

THE TAKE-CHARGE APPROACH helps people to develop confidence in their ability to control and surmount even very severe arthritis symptoms.

By definition, 'chronic' means you have a problem indefinitely or even for life. Arthritis and other chronic illnesses usually develop slowly and then linger. Acute health problems usually run a predictable course of illness followed by healing and cure, but a diagnosis of one of the types of arthritis involves much more uncertainty and many more questions, such as:

◗ Will I have to give up my favourite activities?

◗ Can therapies keep my disease from progressing or help to stabilize it?

◗ Will my pain and disability worsen?

◗ Will additional joints become affected?

◗ Can I continue to provide for my family?

◗ Can I perform the simple activities of everyday life that allow me to stay independent?

◗ How do I deal with the anger and frustration I feel?

◗ How will this affect my relationships with family and friends?

Patient in charge

People with chronic health problems must deal with complex challenges every day. Even as they cope with their condition both medically and surgically, they face tremendous uncertainty about the course of their disease and its impact on their lives. Add these burdens to the pain and disability caused by the chronic illness itself, and patients can become frustrated and depressed.

Clearly, the key ingredient in managing a chronic condition is the patient's own involvement in making the decisions about his or her care.

Passive to aggressive This need for patients to participate in their own health care may seem obvious now. But until quite recently, most patients with chronic health problems took a passive approach to treatment. They went to the doctor to find out how they were doing and rarely asked questions. If a drug was not helping or was causing stomach pain or some other adverse effect, they would rarely complain. After all, who were they to question the doctor's wisdom or to judge whether a treatment was working?

> ● **FACT** Always use the strongest and largest joints and muscles for the job. Getting up from a chair can place a great deal of strain on your hands if you push yourself with your fingertips. Instead of using your fingers or knuckles, use your palms to help you to achieve lift-off.

Accentuate the positive

You may be familiar with Norman Vincent Peale's book, *The Power of Positive Thinking*. The take-charge approach to arthritis emphasizes something similar – the power of a positive attitude. Studies have shown that when people adopt a take-charge attitude toward their arthritis, this positive approach can do wonders for their pain control and degree of disability.

'Because of its chronic nature, arthritis patients must learn to manage and cope with the disease on a day-to-day basis. Their ability to succeed in this task commonly differentiates those who are incapacitated from those who continue to lead full and active lives...'

– Kate Lorig and Halsted Holman, arthritis self-management studies

The **'Challenging Arthritis' course** This self-management programme is based on the work which was developed by Stanford University in 1979. Arthritis Care in the UK started running the courses at the end of 1993 and then extended them, nationwide, a year later. By 2002 there were nearly 200 courses catering for 2,500 people with arthritis, in the UK.

Challenging Arthritis (CA) is designed to enable people with arthritis to manage their lives more effectively and to give them new attitudes and approaches to life.

Although many people who have done the course in the UK started out having doubts, they are usually enthusiastic about the benefits. The course helps them to make sense of what has happened to them and to think through new possibilities. The course is always delivered by people with arthritis, who have been trained by Arthritis Care, and course leaders are carefully supervised to make sure they are working well. There is one session a week for six weeks, and each session lasts for about two and a half hours, including breaks.

Acquired optimism Throughout the six weeks, participants learn more about their arthritis and the factors that can help to control it, including diet, exercise, better pacing, assertiveness and coping with depression and fatigue. These new coping skills are practised and perfected with the mutual support of other course members.

The courses are always held in a community setting, such as a church, village or school hall. Arthritis Care believes that this works better, gearing the programme towards creating a pro-active partnership rather than being seen as the course taking over the treatment of the members' arthritis. Arthritis Care makes sure that members understand that their course is not a substitute for medical treatment; it participates actively with health professionals, and complements and supplements the treatment they are giving to arthritis sufferers.

The Challenging Arthritis course involves looking at life skills, such as how to go about visiting the rheumatologist – what questions to ask, for instance. The organizers like to think that participants on the course go away with a tool-box of life skills. Not all of the tools will be needed all of the time, but it is good to know they're there. Flare-ups occur with arthritis, and it is useful to be able to dip into that tool-box to select the tool that will get you through the crisis.

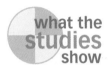

what the **studies** show

▶ In 2000, a study was conducted by Professor Julie Barlow, at the University of Coventry, into the effectiveness of the Challenging Arthritis course. Not only did it find that people were experiencing long-term benefits from having been on the course, but that visits to the GP for pain relief had decreased – so the NHS was benefiting from their improved health, too, in terms of freeing GPs to see other patients, and saving on prescriptions.

The course that changes lives

In studies of people who had enrolled in the Challenging Arthritis courses, researchers found that the positive attitude gained by participants produced other results, too:

1 Four months after completing the course, participants were continuing with strengthening and relaxation exercises, and showed a decrease in fatigue, anxiety and depression. They were aware of better communication skills, especially with their doctors.

2 The beneficial effects from participating in the course lasted. A year later, participants were still following the exercise routines, and benefiting from decreased levels of fatigue, anxiety and depression. In addition, there was a significant decrease in pain and fewer visits to the doctor.

Measure your take-charge quotient

The developers of Stanford University's arthritis self-management programme created a test to help people assess their confidence in handling the consequences of their condition – a concept referred to as the TQ (take-charge quotient). Assessing your TQ regularly can provide you with an ongoing estimate of how you are coping with and taking charge of your own arthritis.

Take a few minutes to answer the questions in the next three sections, which measure your TQ for pain, functioning and 'other symptoms', and then work out your score. A low TQ score (between 10 and 60) in one or more areas means that you could benefit from adopting a take-charge attitude. Once you are working on your own self-management programme, doing the test again will help you to assess your progress.

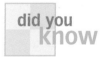
did you know

▶ Pain reduction from taking the arthritis self-help course is almost the same as the decrease in pain achieved by the use of nonsteroidal anti-inflammatory drugs – and is greater than the pain relief from medical or surgical treatments that patients receive.

Pain TQ

On a scale of 10 (very uncertain) to 100 (very certain):

1 How certain are you that you can significantly decrease your pain?

2 How certain are you that you can continue most of your daily activities?

3 How certain are you that you can keep arthritis pain from interfering with your sleep?

4 How certain are you that you can achieve a small to moderate reduction in your arthritis pain by using methods other than taking extra medication?

5 How certain are you that you can make a large reduction in your arthritis pain by using methods other than taking extra medication?

To get an average of your scores for questions 1 to 5, add the scores and divide the total by 5. This will give you your Pain TQ.

Functioning TQ

On a scale of 10 (very uncertain) to 100 (very certain), how sure are you at this moment that you can:

1 Walk 30 yards on flat ground in 20 seconds?

2 Walk 10 steps downstairs in seven seconds?

3 Get out of an armless chair quickly, without using your hands for support?

4 Button and unbutton three medium-size buttons in a row in 12 seconds?

5 Cut two bite-sized pieces of meat with a knife and fork in eight seconds?

6 Turn a garden tap all the way on and all the way off?

7 Scratch your upper back with both your right and left hands?

8 Get in and out of the passenger side of a car without help from another person and without physical aids?

9 Put on a long-sleeved front-opening shirt or blouse (without buttoning) in eight seconds?

To take an average of your scores for questions 1 to 9, add your scores and divide the total by 9. This will give you your Functioning TQ.

Arthritis profile

William Ernest Henley

Few people illustrate triumph over adversity better than William Ernest Henley. He was born in Gloucester in 1849. At the age of 12 he was diagnosed with tubercular arthritis, a crippling and painful condition, and when he was 16 doctors amputated his left leg below the knee.

Henley went on to finish his schooling and became a successful journalist in London. But at 24, threatened with the loss of his other leg to tuberculosis, Henley went to Edinburgh and put himself under the care of the physician Joseph Lister, who managed to save the leg.

During his long hospital stay, Henley wrote *Invictus*. The poem's theme of self-reliance in the face of overwhelming odds has inspired many people.

Invictus

Out of the night that covers me
Black as the Pit from pole to pole,
I thank whatever gods may be
For my unconquerable soul.

In the fell clutch of circumstance
I have not winced nor cried aloud;
Under the bludgeonings of chance
My head is bloody, but unbowed.

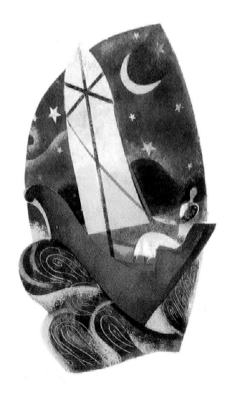

Beyond this place of wrath and tears
Looms but the Horror of the shade,
And yet the menace of the years
Finds, and shall find, me unafraid.

It matters not how strait the gate,
How charged with punishments the scroll,
I am the master of my fate:
I am the captain of my soul.

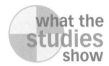

what the studies show

● Among more than 1,000 women, aged 65 and over, who were participating in a women's health and ageing study in Baltimore, Maryland, 115 reported that a doctor had diagnosed them with rheumatoid arthritis. But doctors at the Johns Hopkins Geriatric Center in Baltimore could verify the diagnosis in only 21 per cent of these women. In describing their findings in the June 2000 issue of *The Journal of Rheumatology*, the doctors noted that women taking arthritis medication were especially likely to believe – mistakenly – that they had rheumatoid arthritis. The doctors also found that seven women who failed to report having rheumatoid arthritis did, in fact, have the disease.

'Other symptoms' TQ

On a scale of 10 (very uncertain) to 100 (very certain):

1 How certain are you that you can control your fatigue?

2 How certain are you that you can regulate your activity so as to be active without aggravating your arthritis?

3 How certain are you that you can do something to help yourself feel better if you are feeling blue?

4 As compared with other people with arthritis like yours, how certain are you that you can manage arthritis pain during your daily activities?

5 How certain are you that you can manage your arthritis symptoms so that you can do the things you enjoy doing?

6 How certain are you that you can deal with the frustration of arthritis?

Take the average of your scores for questions 1 to 6 by adding them and dividing the total by 6 to calculate your 'Other symptoms' TQ. Compare all three TQs regularly, to assess your progress.

What does taking charge mean?

Having a chronic disease like arthritis means that, probably, a total cure is not possible. In all likelihood, you will have arthritis for the rest of your life, so you will have to manage the problem one way or another – the choice is up to you.

One unfortunate but all-too-common reaction to a chronic disease is simply to resign oneself to it, a condition psychologists refer to as learned helplessness. A slightly better management style is to merely do whatever your doctor tells you to do. The best approach of all – the approach most likely to ease your pain, improve your mobility, and allow you to live life to the fullest – is to manage your arthritis in a positive way: in short, to take charge of it.

Become the manager of your health Taking charge of your arthritis is not that much different from being a manager in the business world. For example, most top managers rely on consultants when making a decision. In your case, the consultants will include family members and friends and, of course, health-care professionals including your physician, pharmacist or physiotherapist. But ultimately, all they can really offer you is advice. Since you are the manager of your arthritis, it's up to you to put their recommendations into action.

However, arthritis self-help courses, though often useful, are not necessarily right for everyone, and you may not want to follow the eight-step programme we describe. If you're not a programme person, you may find that pursuing just a few of the steps – getting to know your problem, for example, or thinking about your long-term goals – can make a significant difference to the way you feel.

Becoming a skilled patient

Because you are a take-charge person, or intend to become one, you need to equip yourself with the tools that have been proven to ease symptoms: exercises and drugs to reduce pain, helpful devices and surgical techniques for improving mobility, as well as visualization techniques for improving your mood – and many others. But to get the most out of each of them, you need to become a skilled patient.

Once you have learned and mastered the following eight steps, you'll be well on your way to controlling your arthritis, now and in the future, as well as during the inevitable ups and downs you may confront as your symptoms wax and wane.

Getting acquainted with your pain

A big part of getting to know your arthritis problem is gaining a better understanding of how pain affects your life. One way to do that is to keep a pain diary.

About three times a day, pause in your activities, assess your pain, and write down your observations. On a scale of 0 (no pain) to 10 (the worst pain you've ever had), how bad is the pain right now? What is its character – throbbing, burning, aching, stabbing? How does the pain make you feel emotionally – frustrated, hopeless, angry?

Also, jot down what you were doing when you stopped to fill in your diary, and what you did to relieve the pain.

1 Get to know your problem

Studies show that the better arthritis patients understand their disease, the more likely they are to overcome it. You may think you're already quite knowledgable about your condition, especially if you've had it a while. Having lived with something for many years – whether it's a son, a daughter or a disease – might lead you to assume that you're intimately familiar with it.

But what you think you know about your arthritis – what has caused it, how to treat it or prevent it from worsening – may not be true, or may be based on outdated information. In fact, you may not even have the disease you think you have. Even if your symptoms resemble those of your relative or neighbour, you may have an entirely different type of arthritis – or a health problem that isn't even arthritis.

Get a proper diagnosis Receiving a diagnosis of arthritis certainly is not welcome news. But at least you now know the cause of your pain, stiffness or disability. Armed with that knowledge, you can take the first steps towards overcoming the disease and its symptoms.

So, if you haven't already done so, your first step in taking charge of your condition should be to get a definitive diagnosis of your problem. If you are unsure about what type of arthritis you have – or even whether you have it – make an appointment with a doctor, who can evaluate you. Chapter 4 (*Working with your doctor*) tells you about the physicians who are qualified to diagnose arthritis.

Once you're sure about what type of arthritis you have, Chapter 2 (*Know your arthritis*) can help you to become an expert on it. The chapter takes you inside the joints where problems arise and offers you comprehensive descriptions of the major arthritic conditions: osteoarthritis, rheumatoid arthritis and fibromyalgia, as well as less common but important ailments such as gout and lupus. You will also see the latest findings on causes, diagnostic techniques and treatments.

One patient's learning curve

Consider the case of Jim, a 60-year-old grandfather living in the USA. Recently, Jim realized that the twinge he had first noticed in his left knee a few years ago had become much worse. The knee was stiff for a good 15 or 20 minutes after he got out of bed in the morning. Walking for more than a block or so caused sharp, intermittent pain. Jim had always prided himself on being physically active, yet now his painful knee was preventing him from doing the things he loved – from playing catch with his grandson to going bird-watching with his wife.

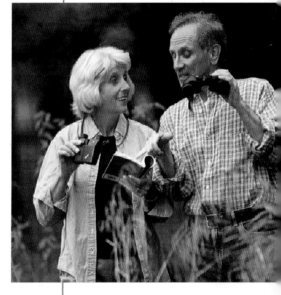

Jim regretted having to withdraw from the activities that had brought him joy. But he accepted that aches, pains and stiffness were a normal part of getting older – something he would just have to live with.

What the doctor discovered Jim's wife, however, had noticed that her husband was becoming increasingly depressed as his knee problems worsened. She urged him to find out whether anything could be done. So Jim made an appointment with a rheumatologist, a doctor who specializes in treating arthritis and related conditions that affect the joints.

After taking Jim's history and doing a physical examination, the doctor told him that he had osteoarthritis of the knee. But he tempered the diagnosis with some good news: many treatment options were available – not only for preventing the pain and stiffness in his knee from worsening, but also for reducing the symptoms and giving Jim back his active life.

Jim made a second appointment with the rheumatologist to discuss his condition and his possible treatment options in more detail. In the meantime, he began reading about the strategy outlined in this book in order to learn more about the causes of osteoarthritis and the take-charge approach for gaining control

2 Choose your long-term goal

People diagnosed with arthritis have a wide range of goals, from the unrealistic ('I want to be cured') to the vague ('I want to feel better') to the specific and realistic ('I want to climb the stairs unaided'). Specific, realistic goals are best.

How to be goal-oriented

Dr. Margaret A. Caudill, Ph.D., a leading pain specialist at Harvard University and New England Deaconess Hospital in Boston, says that every self-management goal should be:

Measurable Define it in numerical terms if possible.
Wrong I'll develop better sleeping habits.
Right I will go to bed by 10 on most nights.

Realistic Can you meet it, even if you are having pain?
Wrong I will catch up on my work without getting tired and hurting.
Right I will stretch and do hand-relaxing exercises for five minutes every hour.

Behavioural It should be a specific action that you can take.
Wrong I will be more upbeat.
Right Whenever I feel hopeless, I will do a relaxation exercise and redirect my thoughts.

'I'-centred Make it something that *you* personally will do.
Wrong Everyone will give me time for my shower.
Right I will take a hot shower every morning.

Desirable Is the effort worth the reward?
There is no right or wrong way here; just pay attention to yourself and act accordingly.

GOALS

1 _____

2 _____

3 _____

4 _____

In fact, you will learn that the take-charge approach to arthritis is based on setting and attaining specific goals. For one thing, you can readily tell whether or not you have attained a specific goal. You'll also find it's easier to motivate yourself to reach a specific goal than one that is vague or perhaps even undefinable.

Spend a few minutes thinking about your goals, and write them down on the lines above. Try to list your goals in their order of importance to you, and try to choose goals that are measurable. Your most important goal is the one you should work towards first.

Before Jim's next appointment with his rheumatologist, he sat down to write out his goals. He tried to think of changes that would be especially valuable in transforming his life. He soon realized that one goal – walking a relatively long distance without knee pain – held the key to achieving several other goals. It also had the virtue of being measurable and realistic. So he listed this as his number-one goal, along with several others:

1 Be able to walk a mile without knee pain
2 Go bird-watching with my wife, Sharon
3 Play catch with my grandson, Sean
4 Work in the garden again

3 Decide on a strategy

Now that you have chosen your goals, it's time to formulate your arthritis strategy – that is, in treatment terms, the options you have for achieving those goals.

Learning to pick and choose In devising their strategy, arthritis patients obviously have many approaches to choose from. Arthritis often responds to some form of drug treatment. Alternative approaches, such as dietary supplements or perhaps mind-body treatments, also do the trick for some patients. Exercise helps most types of arthritis; surgery is an option when disability is severe.

As the manager of your arthritis, you should select the approaches that have the best chance of being successful for you. You may want a strategy that combines several different approaches, all of which may help you to attain your long-term goal. Even if one approach is only modestly successful, others may prove more effective.

Think strategically

With your goals in mind, think about the treatment approaches that might help you to attain them. Reading the later chapters in this book can help you to choose the approaches best suited to you and your condition.

As the manager of your own arthritis, feel free to consult other people as you narrow down your list of treatment options to one or more that have the best chance of resulting in success. Your doctor, family members and friends may all have opinions on approaches that are most likely to work for you. However, just remember that you are the one who should have the final say on the treatments you use.

Treatments you'll stick with Try to choose the sorts of treatment that you like well enough to tolerate long term. If you've always hated exercise, don't make it one of your treatment

APPROACHES

1 _____

2 _____

3 _____

4 _____

options. You may be more enthusiastic about a less physical approach that includes relaxation, guided imagery or other mind-body techniques.

Once you've decided on some possible approaches, write them on the lines at the bottom of page 104. Try to list them in the order in which you'd be most likely to use them.

Jim chooses his strategy

Jim learned about a number of possible options for treating osteoarthritis of the knee. He wrote down four that particularly appealed to him and discussed them with his rheumatologist at his next appointment:

1 Take pain-relieving drugs

2 Lose 10lb

3 Strengthen quadriceps muscles

4 Get hyaluronic-acid injections in the knee

Now it was time to look at those strategies. Which of them would be best for reaching his goal of walking a mile without pain? Together, Jim and his doctor reviewed the benefits and drawbacks of the various options that Jim had selected.

Take pain-relieving drugs Jim had learned that the recently introduced COX-2 pain relievers (Celebrex, Vioxx or Mobic) pose lower risk of stomach upset than standard NSAIDs such as ibuprofen – a really important consideration for him. But because Jim had an active stomach ulcer, his doctor advised him against using any type of NSAID, including the COX-2s. So Jim eliminated drug treatment as a strategy.

Lose 10lb Jim had been overweight since he was a teenager. He knew that shedding excess pounds can do much to alleviate knee pain. His doctor agreed that losing 10lb could be a useful strategy for Jim.

Strengthen quadriceps muscles Jim already knew that arthritic knee pain responds well to exercises that strengthen the quadriceps (thigh) muscles. Jim and his doctor reviewed several

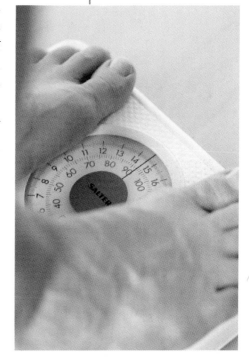

exercises which specifically target the quadriceps muscles. The doctor also recommended two other exercises for strengthening Jim's leg muscles – regular walking and using an exercise bicycle. Walking and pedalling would improve Jim's aerobic conditioning and also help in his weight-loss efforts by burning calories.

Get hyaluronic-acid injections in the knee Jim knew that these shots offered the potential of reduced knee pain. But Jim's doctor noted that some rheumatologists were still not convinced about the usefulness of the injections – which, in any case, were expensive (three to five injections cost about £180 in the UK). Jim decided against the injections.

In the end, Jim decided to focus on two treatment approaches to relieve his knee pain – losing 10lb and strengthening his quadriceps muscles. Now that he had defined his arthritis strategy, it was time to pursue his goal in a systematic way.

4 Draw up your weekly take-charge plan

Take-charge planning is a means of reaching your ultimate goal through a succession of short-term goals. Think of the plan as a weekly contract that you make with yourself. Each week you assign yourself a series of specific actions, then build on your accomplishments from week to week. Ideally, someone who could climb only five stairs at week one will be climbing three flights after several weeks.

> ◗ **FACT** Buying a daily planner in which you schedule all of your activities – including rest periods – will help you to keep on track.

Making the commitment Being committed to a personal plan may seem a bit of a burden at first. But once you get into the habit, you will find that it is well worth the effort. Your weekly successes will help to convince you that you can indeed take charge of your arthritis and overcome the restrictions that the disease has imposed on you.

In creating your weekly plan, you will have to take active steps to implement your personal approach to treatment. So if you have decided on a weight-loss approach, your plan will include weight-loss strategies such as eliminating between-meal snacks or walking to burn up calories. Shopping carefully for food will help – don't be tempted to put fattening snacks into the trolley.

Success is in the detail The key to a successful plan is to make your strategies very specific (so they will be easier to repeat) and measurable (so you can easily score your success in completing them). If 'walking' is one of them, for example, you should specify when you intend to walk ('before breakfast'), where ('around the block'), how often ('Monday, Wednesday and Friday'), for how long ('10 minutes').

If you make your plan too ambitious, you may become discouraged by failure. On the other hand, you won't make progress if your plan is too modest. Ideally, try to include actions that are achievable but that may require a little effort. Once you've achieved them, you can write in slightly more ambitious strategies for next week's plan.

Jim makes a plan

Jim's weekly take-charge plan incorporated both of his treatment strategies – losing weight and exercising. Since Jim had been a confirmed couch potato, his doctor gave him some good advice: 'Set modest short-term goals during the first week. Perform each action just a few times, for just a few minutes, or at low intensity.

did you know

▶ Moving around a bit at least every two hours can fend off stiffness. If you are inclined to sit too much, go out for a walk. If you must stand for a prolonged time, enjoy a few moments off your feet. Set an alarm clock to remind you to take your breaks, if you're likely to forget.

Plan	Day	Action	Where	Time	Results
	Monday	Leg flexes	Bedroom	Before work	✔
		Stationary bike	Fitness club	After work	✔
	Tuesday	Walk around the block	Sheridan Park	Lunchtime	✔
	Wednesday	Leg flexes	Bedroom	Before work	✔
		Stationary bike	Fitness club	After work	–
	Thursday	Walk around the block	Sheridan Park	Lunchtime	✔
	Friday	Leg flexes	Bedroom	Before work	–
		Stationary bike	Fitness club	After work	✔
	Saturday	–	–	–	
	Sunday	–	–	–	

You'll have ample opportunity to make things more strenuous in the coming weeks, as your body adjusts to exercise.'

Together with his doctor, Jim settled on three very specific activities for his first week. He would do some more often than others. His take-charge plan for exercise is on the previous page.

Your weekly take-charge plan In writing up your weekly take-charge plan, be as specific as possible. State what you plan to do, how much you intend to do, when and where you will do these activities and how many days a week you'll do them.

Plan

Day	Action	Where	Time	Results
Monday				
Tuesday				
Wednesday				
Thursday				
Friday				
Saturday				
Sunday				

5 Put your take-charge plan into action

Now comes the hard part – sticking to the weekly plan that you've devised. Be prepared to do some work, and perhaps even make some sacrifices; nothing worthwhile comes easily.

Jim springs into action

Jim found that setting aside time to exercise several days a week wasn't easy. As for the challenges of his weight-loss approach, he had a very hard time giving up the luxury ice cream he was accustomed to having after dinner every night.

> ⊙ **FACT** If you haven't exercised in a while and are apprehensive about taking the plunge, consult an expert. A physician who specializes in rehabilitative medicine or a physiotherapist can help you to design an exercise programme to suit your physical condition and your goals.

Jim found that taking charge of his arthritis meant first taking charge of himself and adjusting the way he had been living. 'Old habits die hard', the saying goes, and adopting new ones can be even harder. Jim discovered that changing his old habits and forming new ones took persistence, but was worth the effort.

How Jim changed Jim had to wean himself off some of his favourite television shows in order to fit in his exercise sessions. But he didn't have to give up TV completely – he simply taped the shows and watched them later. And when it came to giving up his full-fat ice cream fix, he down-graded into lower-fat varieties for several months and then, as his tastebuds became used to the 'thinner' taste, moved into fat-free brands. He also trained himself to eat slightly less.

Jim also learned to be patient. His arthritis didn't develop overnight, so he realized that he shouldn't expect rapid improvement, either. It took him time to master the necessary skills. And even after he put his take-charge plan into practice,

'I hated contracting when I took the self-help course. But now, as a course leader, I see that contracting is what changes people the most. It helps them find for the first time that they have control over their arthritis and can do things they never expected.'

– Sharon Dorough, arthritis self-help course leader

it took several weeks before he started noticing improvements. However, he eventually attained those goals that he wished for and which had been previously out of reach.

Getting started

How many actions should you pack into your weekly plan, how often should you do them and how much effort should you expend on them? The best advice is to take things quite slowly and easily, especially to start with.

How many actions? Plan just one or two activities for your first week. Beginning with just a couple increases your chances of sticking to your assignment and of your weekly take-charge plan developing into a habit. If you find yourself failing, you are more likely to give up altogether.

How often will you do them? Doing something every day can be tedious as well as tiring. Probably the best frequency for any action is three to four times a week. The one exception is medication, which may need to be taken every day.

> **◗ FACT** It can take time to assess how well a drug is relieving pain. NSAIDs require a one or two-week trial to see if they work; slower-acting drugs such as gold (injected or in tablet form) may require six months.

How much will you do? Take your present condition as your starting point and progress gradually from there. If your knees start to hurt after you walk one block, your first plan should not call for walking a mile. On the other hand, you don't want to be so conservative that you don't make progress. As with so much in life, moderation is the best policy.

6 Monitor your progress

As you follow your take-charge plan during the week, gauge whether you've met each day's goals. You can do that directly by checking off the actions you have completed. Closely following up in this way gives you rapid and helpful feedback.

You should congratulate yourself if you've conscientiously stuck with the plan. But don't be hard on yourself if you have scored some 'incompletes'. Instead, write out the same take-charge plan for the following week and see if you can do better.

Making progress, inch by inch You may not be able to detect progress on a day-to-day basis, but an effective plan should produce small improvements each week. How do you assess such progress? You need to step back a bit and regularly take stock of how you're doing. Look at the TQ tests (pages 95-98). Using them, you can assess whether your efforts are making a difference – that they are moving you steadily toward your goal. Another way to do this is through the use of 'progress points'.

Progress points: useful milestones

In carrying out the activities in your take-charge plan, such as 'walk around the block for a half hour before dinner each night', for example, you achieve the short-term goals that you want to build on, week by week.

Unfortunately, meeting your short-term goals does not mean you are making progress from week to week. You may feel that you're moving forward when, in fact, you're running on the spot. Using progress points can help to overcome this problem. They tell you whether your combined actions are working and you are on course with your weekly actions.

Jim takes stock Jim's take-charge plan incorporates a weight-loss approach. According to experts, losing 1lb a week is a reasonable weight-loss goal for overweight people. Now Jim has a progress point – 'lose 1lb this week' – which helps him to measure how well he is doing so that he can decide how strenuous his weight-loss actions should be.

You can lose one pound a week by using up 3,500 more calories than you take in. So Jim's plan might consist of a low-fat diet and fat-burning exercises that, taken together, make a 3,500 calorie difference. Simply by weighing himself at the end of the week, Jim is able to monitor his progress and the success of his plan.

> **caution**
>
> Don't over-exert yourself if your take-charge plan involves exercise. To keep exertion within safe limits, exercise at an intensity that allows you to speak without gasping for air.

7 Adjust your action plan

If at first you don't succeed . . . maybe it's time to redo your plan. Perhaps your short-term goals are too ambitious and you need to scale back or allow yourself more time for completing them. With progress points you can gauge whether your take-charge plan needs to be adjusted.

If your progress point called for losing 1lb last week and you lost only 8oz, perhaps you need to intensify your actions. If you lost more than 1lb, maybe you're working too hard and need to moderate your activities. Either way, your progress point tells you that you need to fine-tune your plan.

Jim makes adjustments

Sometimes the best progress point is how you feel. Jim's plan called for doing two sets of leg flexes to help strengthen the muscles around his knee. At the end of the first week, his thigh muscles were very sore.

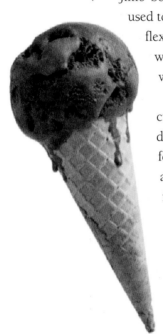

Jim's body was obviously sending him a message: 'I'm not used to this much exertion.' So he decided to reduce his leg-flex regimen from two sets to one for the following two weeks. After that, if he experienced no muscle pain, Jim would try to resume doing two sets of leg flexes a day.

Jim also found that the transition from low-fat ice cream to virtually fat-free was something he couldn't do easily. After a bowl of fat-free cherry vanilla, he still found himself loitering in the kitchen looking for an additional sweet treat to make up for his unsatisfying iced dessert.

So he explored the ice-cream section in his local supermarket and found that several well-known companies made low-fat varieties of iced dessert that were indeed creamier tasting and more palate-pleasing than the virtually fat-free brand he'd been eating. So he switched brands and cut back on the number of scoops he had.

Correcting your course Mid-course corrections of this sort not only help you to move towards your goal but they also sharpen your coping skills. People with arthritis are constantly confronting uncertainty; unfortunately, flare-ups and setbacks are a normal part of the disease. A large part of taking charge of arthritis is becoming skilled at recognizing problems and then working around them.

◗ **FACT** If you have arthritis of the hands, stock up on pain relievers and vitamins without a child-proof cap. These caps can be hard to open for arthritis sufferers.

If you are a typist, for example, and morning stiffness in your fingers is interfering with your work, the best solution may be to modify your activities: arrange to start your workday later, for example, or build in frequent and regular breaks. Learning to adjust your plan as necessary can help you to develop the flexibility needed to take charge of your arthritis.

8 Building on your success

In a way, building on success is the secret to gaining control over your arthritis. The take-charge approach hinges on achieving small successes week by week – until you arrive at an ultimate goal that may at first have seemed out of reach.

This time-tested formula helps to explain why people who develop a successful plan for themselves tend to stick with it. The success you achieve one week has a beneficial effect not only on your joints but also on your attitude – helping you to build confidence in your ability to manage your disease and to overcome its limitations.

Little victories

Build rewards into your plan, so that obtaining those rewards requires that you successfully complete an action. For example, Jim loved to buy his daily newspaper during his lunch hour. So when he designed his daily lunch-hour walk, he made sure that it took him past a newsstand. For Jim, buying a newspaper was his way of rewarding himself for successfully completing that daily walk.

A final suggestion: give yourself some time off for good behaviour. Focusing on your arthritis every day may seem praiseworthy but can prove thoroughly wearing. You'll have a much greater chance of reaching your goals if you give yourself a day or two off every week.

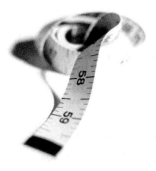

4

Working with your doctor

Many doctors today welcome

their patients' input into treatment

decisions. This is especially

true for doctors who treat chronic

diseases such as arthritis,

for which there is no standard

treatment or cure.

Doctor as advocate

Although many doctors no longer consider themselves all-knowing authorities – a result of the new doctor-patient relationship that has evolved during the past few years – doctors' actions may still be at odds with their intentions. Some recent studies have found that conversations between doctor and patient are often more like lectures than joint efforts to agree on a course of treatment.

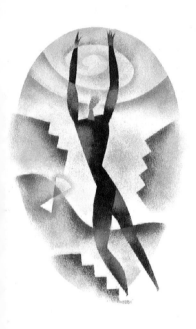

YOU ARE THE MANAGER OF YOUR ARTHRITIS
You enlist the experts – the physicians and other healthcare members – listen to their treatment recommendations and make a shared decision on the course of action that is best for you.

Be assertive Clearly, there is a need for patients to be assertive in their dealings with doctors. For you, that means being well informed and actively participating in your interactions with your GP, rheumatologist and the other healthcare professionals involved in your care. It encompasses:

❍ Deciding whether you could benefit from seeing your GP in the first place

❍ Choosing a GP whose expertise and personality meet your needs

❍ Understanding why your GP will need to take a complete medical history during your initial visit

❍ Ensuring you get the information you need in the limited time available in your GP appointment

❍ Knowing how other healthcare professionals can help you to overcome your illness and improve your quality of life

As you work with the members of your healthcare team, remember that you are the most important person involved in your treatment. Having taken charge of your arthritis, you are not putting yourself 'under the care' of anyone. Instead, you are the manager of your arthritis and, in fact, you will be the one carrying out the mutually agreed upon treatment plans.

Strategies for communicating with your doctor

1 Make eye contact. Wait until you can make eye contact before you start talking about your problem. Doctors are frequently preoccupied with the unavoidable trappings of modern medicine – notes, computers and reference materials.

2 Go from general statements to specific statements. Doctors have been taught to think this way.

3 Go from subjective (what you feel) to objective (information you can see, count or touch). Your doctor's thought pattern is also moving in this way.

4 Always explain how your problems affect your life, work, relationships, sleep, etc. This is the most powerful way of illustrating the impact arthritis is having on you. It will help to elicit your doctor's compassion and serve as a reminder that a person, not just a disease, is being treated.

5 Pause between parts of your story. This will allow your doctor to take notes and ask questions.

—From *Don't Let Your HMO Kill You* (a book about US health maintenance organizations)

Do you even need a doctor?

For people severely affected by arthritis, or diagnosed with a type (such as RA) that must be carefully monitored, the answer is clearly yes: they need to see their GPs and take the drugs that only doctors can prescribe to ease symptoms and prevent joint damage from worsening.

But for other people with arthritis – perhaps even the majority – whose symptoms are mild and manageable, the decision about whether to consult a doctor isn't so obvious. For them, the take-charge approach – emphasizing self-care actions such as weight

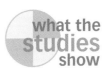
what the studies show

▷ A study of consultations found that doctors allow patients to talk for an average of only 18 seconds before interrupting them – and then spend less than 2 minutes of a 20 minute session sharing information with patients.

loss and exercise – may provide all the benefits they've been seeking. Or perhaps they did see a doctor years ago and have successfully followed through on the advice they received.

Doctor to the rescue Some patients who have decided against seeing a doctor could genuinely benefit from it. Sometimes their opposition stems from ignorance of their disease or of treatments that are available. But all too often, such patients have a defeatist attitude towards their condition. They believe that it will inevitably worsen and so they must simply endure the accompanying pain and disability.

Facing the fears of arthritis

Some arthritis patients let fear rule their lives – as well as the management of their condition – when confronting it would help them to progress to the next step of treatment or even to build a supportive healthcare team. Here are three common fears along with strategies to put them into perspective:

Fear of the unknown It is up to you, as we've already said, to educate yourself about your condition, ask questions of your doctor, and move into the daylight of enlightenment about your particular type of arthritis.

Fear of medication It's a fact that all medications can cause side effects. Once again, knowing which medication works best for you, with minimum side effects, is the best defence against this fear. Every person responds differently to the same drug. Ask your doctor or pharmacist about the drug – and read up on your own – so that you are comfortable with the choice of medication you and your doctor have made.

Fear of depending on others On one hand, you should actively pursue good nutrition, physical therapy and other alternatives to help to maintain your independence. On the other hand, your friends and family should be part of your health-care team. Your family will understand your suffering as no one else will. Share your thoughts and fears with them, and they can help you work toward solutions.

Since arthritis is rarely fatal, this misplaced stoicism usually isn't life-threatening. But by missing out on effective treatments, people may be subjecting themselves to needless pain and suffering. In addition, this neglect of their condition may allow joint damage to progress to the point that it can no longer be reversed except by surgery.

Should I see a doctor? The answer certainly is 'yes' if you are experiencing one or more of the following symptoms:

- Persistent pain or stiffness after getting out of bed in the morning

- Soreness and swelling in any joint or in a symmetrical pair of joints (both sides of the body)

- Recurrence of the above symptoms, especially when more than one joint is involved

- Recurrent or persistent pain and stiffness in the neck, lower back, knees and other joints

- Loss of weight, fatigue and fever accompanied by joint pain

In addition, there are other, more general reasons to consider seeing a doctor:

- If problems with your joints are interfering with your daily life and your normal activities

- If you find yourself avoiding activities that you've previously loved doing

- If your joint pain is interfering with sleep

- If you find you are avoiding shopping or other social activities because you don't want to 'slow everybody else down' and draw attention to your limitations

- If the pain in your joints or the limitations it imposes on your physical activities are begining to make you feel anxious, helpless or depressed

did you know

Pulled muscles, bone bruises and ligament and other injuries can mimic the pain of osteoarthritis.

In the spirit of taking charge of your arthritis, it may be time to make an appointment with your GP. Remember, you are under no obligation to agree with his or her recommendations. But it is quite possible that you will find that working with your GP may provide the crucial missing ingredient that will make your take-charge programme a success.

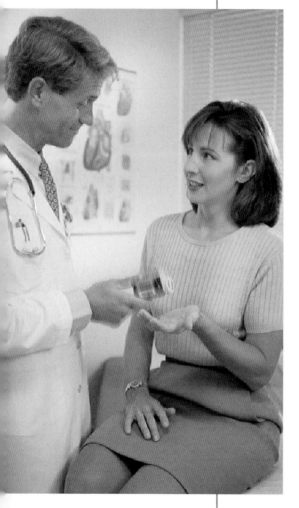

The medical marriage: how to tie the knot

For many common medical problems, such as the inevitable colds, allergies, earaches, cuts and scrapes, our contact with doctors is episodic and usually brief: perhaps an initial appointment and maybe a follow-up visit. Arthritis, on the other hand, is a chronic health problem, which means that a different treatment approach is needed.

Patients with arthritis may need regular and sometimes frequent consultations over a period of years, to monitor the patient's overall physical and emotional health, to check for possible side effects from potent prescription drugs, and to deal with flare-ups as they arise. Perhaps most crucially, there is no one 'correct treatment' for a chronic disease like arthritis. As a result, managing a patient's disease may involve trying first one treatment, then another, or perhaps using several in combination.

○ FACT The patient's words are of key importance when talking to a doctor. Studies have shown that between 60 and 70 per cent of all the information doctors need for diagnosis comes from the patient's medical history – an explanation of the medical problem in the patient's own words.

Symptom sorting

There is an art to telling your doctor about symptoms, when it comes to arthritis. Saying your knee hurts won't shed much light on your problem. Whenever possible, be specific.

For instance:

- How long the joint has felt painful or stiff

- What the pain is like, for example, constant or intermittent, or burning, throbbing, aching or stabbing

- How the pain or stiffness has evolved, for example, mild at first and then increasingly severe, or severe from the very beginning

- What time of day the pain or stiffness is worse

- What makes the pain or stiffness in the joint feel better or worse

- How long the joint feels stiff after you get up in the morning

- Whether the joint symptoms were preceded by illness or seemed to occur spontaneously

- How the symptoms are affecting your life, for example, do they prevent you from performing recreational activities that you've been able to do in the past, and do you feel frustrated or depressed because of this limitation?

List any other symptoms you've been experiencing, even if you don't think they could possibly be related to your condition. These would include fatigue, fever, chills, depression or anxiety.

Are you compatible? Caring for someone with arthritis lends itself to a long-term partnership between patient and doctor. Your treatment may well entail many visits to your GP and the surgery is likely to become familiar territory.

Just like marriage or any other extended relationship, you should feel compatible with the physician you team up with. Whether you do feel comfortable depends as much on the GP's personality as your own.

Some patients thrive on the breezy, light-hearted approach, while others prefer their doctors to be serious and reflective. But there is one 'doctor quality' that is crucially important to all patients – the ability to communicate and explain things clearly. Communication, however, is a two-way street – and you, as the patient, need to work at your side of the relationship.

Know your doctor

When it comes to choosing a doctor to treat your arthritis, you will encounter three kinds – GPs, hospital doctors in specialist training and fully accredited consultant rheumatologists. Although you can choose which GP to register with, there may be little or no choice as to whom you see if you are referred to a specialist by your GP. Hospital doctors in training will often be different individuals at each out-patient appointment, and you may see one as part of a consultant's team, rather than the actual boss. If there is more than one rheumatologist in your area, you may have a choice so you can always discuss this possibility with your GP.

Second opinions: switching to a specialist

The majority of arthritis patients have osteoarthritis. And fortunately, most cases of osteoarthritis are mild enough and uncomplicated enough for a GP to provide adequate care. But if your GP has treated you for more than a year, using a variety of different treatments, and your condition has still not improved significantly, then it's probably time to see a rheumatologist.

A good primary-care physician will respect your desire for a second opinion and should be willing to suggest a rheumatologist for you to see. If not, it may be time to see a different GP.

Diagnosed with osteoarthritis? Ask these questions

◐ What made you conclude that I have osteoarthritis?

◐ Can my symptoms have been caused by other conditions?

◐ If I do have osteoarthritis, is it primary (no identifiable cause) or secondary (as a result of another problem)?

◐ If it is secondary osteoarthritis, what other types of treatment could help to eliminate the cause of the problem?

◐ Is there any joint deformity? If so, please tell me where and to what degree.

◐ Are there any bone spurs? If so, where?

◐ Have I lost range of motion in any of my joints? If so, where?

◐ Which treatment do you recommend? Why?

General Practitioners After medical school, GPs undergo postgraduate training in a variety of hospital disciplines such as paediatrics, gynaecology, orthopaedics and general medicine. It is not possible to cover every specialist discipline in the minimum three years but all will have a basic core of necessary disciplines and will have spent a year in a training practice. GPs learn about health problems that affect all ages.

> ◐ **FACT** Don't always expect reassurance. A doctor won't say, 'It's going to be fine' or 'I'm sure it's nothing' until the prognosis is certain. Doctors don't want to reassure you only to have to break bad news later.

If your arthritis is mild or uncomplicated, the starting point for arthritis care is your GP, who can usually diagnose arthritis based on your medical history, a physical examination, laboratory tests

continued on page 126

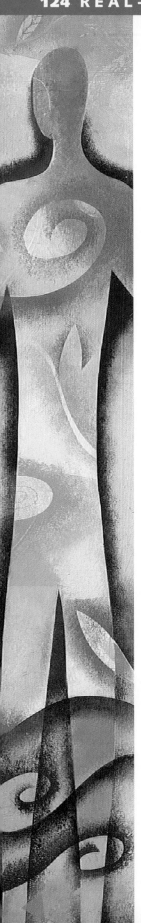

Trust and understanding for best results

Retired headmaster Michael Short has just been playing football in the garden with his granddaughter Rebecca. That's fairly impressive for a 68-year-old, even a fit one, but it is truly amazing for someone with two artificial hips, who had trouble just walking, only a few years ago.

Michael, from Bolton-le-Sands in Lancashire, had always led an active life: he was an accomplished golfer and played three times a week, and also swam three times a week to keep fit. He was also a very keen gardener and really enjoyed getting stuck in to the big tasks.

One day he was lifting some bags of soil that he had bought at the garden centre when suddenly his back went. 'I was in some considerable pain and decided to visit an osteopath to see if he could help,' Michael explains.

The osteopath told Michael his body was tight and felt very tense and rigid. So a course of treatment began, but even after several visits, Michael really felt as if there was no improvement and he decided to stop the treatment. 'I had a feeling there was something wrong with my hips, but I decided to just carry on and live with the pain without doing anything more about it. There seemed no point in making a fuss.'

In the course of the next five years the pain in Michael's legs and hips got worse and worse. 'I'd be trying to do some work in the garden but would end up feeling so much pain that I would have to go and lie down. I just couldn't understand how I could suddenly be like this after previously being so fit,' Michael remembers.

Eventually Michael decided to book an appointment with his local GP. 'My doctor examined me closely and immediately recommended that I have my hips X-rayed.

'Thankfully he also recommended a good specialist for me to see.'

The recommendation was well worthwhile, because looking at the X-rays, the osteopath was able to see immediately that Michael had osteoarthritis.

'The damage to my hips was clear', says Michael, 'and, in fact, was not such a surprise, as my mother had suffered from severe osteoarthritis in her neck.'

It soon appeared that Michael would have to have both hips replaced. A daunting thought, but the decision was made so much easier by the careful handling of the rheumatologist.

'The specialist was wonderfully attentive and explained to me very clearly that surgery would be the best course of action,' says Michael.

But most important of all, Michael's specialist really took the time to clarify the whole procedure involved and made Michael feel and understand that, without any doubt, it was the best course of action.

Michael went in to hospital for the operation to replace his left hip. 'The day after the operation I was out of bed and walking around the ward with the help of a frame' he smiles triumphantly. Twelve days later he left hospital for some serious walking rehabilitation and physiotherapy.

Again, the good advice he received on the importance of rehabilitation was crucial to Michael's recovery. He followed a very careful regime to the letter, and he was able to go back to hospital just three months later for the second hip replacement operation.

Three years have passed since the second operation, and Michael has no regrets whatsoever. 'I can once again enjoy my gardening. I still get tired of course, but that's due more to old age than my new hips. I haven't tried jogging yet but at least I can run across the road when needs be!'

The key to the successful outcome of Michael's two operations was undoubtedly the trust between him and his medical professionals.

'The advice I received was spot-on. Even the nurses looking after me after my operations commented on how the specialist only has one person on his mind during surgery, and that's the patient. It's that sort of dedication and professionalism that gives you the faith to put yourself completely into their hands' says Michael.

In many ways Michael feels fitter than he did ten years ago, 'I'm delighted with the results and unquestionably recommend listening to and following the advice of good professionals.'

> **'I still get tired, of course, but that's due more to old age than my new hips.'**

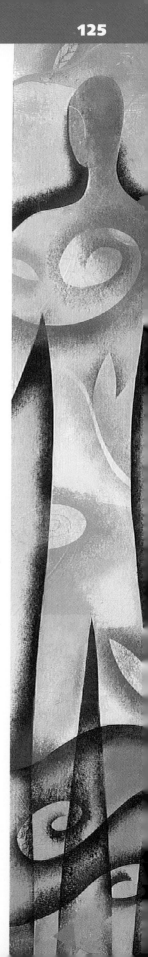

and, sometimes, X-rays. As primary-care physicians, GPs are trained to recognize when a patient's problems are beyond their realm of expertise and require referral to a specialist.

Hospital doctors in specialist training After medical school and a year as a pre-registration house officer, all doctors take another three years of postgraduate training, which emphasizes serious health problems affecting adults. These include disorders of the heart, lungs, gastrointestinal tract, and the endocrine glands – as well as chronic diseases such as arthritis. Some doctors go on to train further in hospital, moving into specific disciplines, and going up the ranks of specialist grades (senior house officer, specialist registrar, senior registrar) while others go into general practice.

Rheumatologists These are physicians who specialize in diagnosing and treating arthritis of all types. They are hospital doctors who have undergone additional years of training in the treatment of arthritis and other problems affecting the joints.

Anyone with any form of inflammatory arthritis, including rheumatoid arthritis, should be referred to a rheumatologist. Rheumatoid arthritis can be a very serious disease and is sometimes even life-threatening. It requires the expertise that only rheumatologists can provide. They are not only knowledgeable about the potent drugs used for treating rheumatoid arthritis but are also experts on their sometimes serious side effects.

▶ **FACT** Osteoarthritis and other forms of arthritis are diagnosed after the pain has been present in a joint for a minimum of two consecutive weeks.

You should also be under the care of a rheumatologist – or at least be referred for a consultation with one – if you have a complicated case of osteoarthritis that requires the use of several drugs. The rheumatologist may be able to devise a treatment plan that makes you feel better than you've thought possible, with fewer side effects.

Your first time:
what to take to the doctor's surgery

By arriving at your initial visit well prepared, you will help your doctor to gain much better insights into your arthritis problems and how they can best be treated. A day or two before your appointment, compile several lists, each of them on a separate piece of paper:

A drug list Your doctor will want to know what drugs you are now taking – not only for your arthritis pain but for any other health problems you may have.

This list can provide insights into your health and will help to prevent the doctor from prescribing medications that might interact with other drugs you are taking.

The list should include prescription drugs, over-the-counter medications such as antacids and pain relievers, and dietary supplements including vitamins, herbs, or any other alternative treatments that you are taking by mouth or rubbing on your skin.

A list of health problems Since a medical history covers past and present health problems, your doctor will probably ask about health problems you have had previously. Make your list as complete as possible, even if it means including ailments you now regard as trivial.

There is a good chance your doctor will also ask about health problems affecting your closest blood relatives (your parents, siblings and children), so include this information as well.

A list of your symptoms During the history, your doctor will ask you to describe your symptoms and then ask you specific questions about them.

By jotting down this information ahead of time – when you don't feel as rushed as you might in the doctor's surgery – you will be able to give your doctor a fuller picture of the extent and severity of your arthritis.

Preparing for the first appointment

Your appointment will provide your GP with basic but vital information about your physical condition. This meeting should help your doctor to sketch out a medical portrait of you and can establish whether you have arthritis and, if so, what type it is.

During the appointment, your GP will take your medical history, asking many questions about your health, and will give you a physical examination. Based on what you say and the examination, the doctor may arrange for you to have X-rays and blood samples taken for laboratory testing. Let's break this appointment down into its components:

The medical history The patient history was traditionally a one-way interrogation, in which the doctor asked questions and the patient answered them. But the modern approach is a more collaborative effort, so feel free to volunteer information that could give your doctor a better insight into your arthritis.

The examination In the physical examination your doctor will examine your joints to see how they function while you're sitting or standing still and when you walk, stretch or bend. It may also include measures such as taking your blood pressure and pulse rate, and listening to your heart.

Closely examining the affected joints, the GP will determine whether they are swollen and, if so, whether the swelling is due to thickened synovial (soft) tissue in the joint (which suggests rheumatoid or some other type of inflammatory arthritis) or is caused by bony swellings (bone spurs indicate that osteoarthritis is present).

Finally, a good diagnostician will look at the pattern of joint involvement: pain or swelling in symmetrical joints (the joints connecting both big toes to the feet, for example) is often a tip-off for rheumatoid arthritis.

X-rays These images can provide objective evidence that arthritis is present – and what type it is. For example, the X-ray images of joints affected by osteoarthritis and rheumatoid arthritis usually look quite different.

what the studies show

▶ Get to the heart of your medical problem quickly. According to one study, patients who were allowed to talk without interruption to their doctor about a problem spoke for 2 minutes. Other research has shown that when a doctor allows a patient to talk for a whole minute, nearly all the information the doctor needs will be revealed. Remember, time is at a premium, with most GP appointments being booked for just 10 minutes, so be as concise as you can.

> ## Physician-patient: one doctor's view
>
> 'It's going to be a long relationship, and neither party should expect too much from the first encounter. A patient's questions should be answered as fully as time allows, and the doctor should expect that the patient will be somewhat anxious.
>
> 'The patient shouldn't expect that the doctor can – or should try to – cover every aspect of the disease and all its possible outcomes during the first visit.
>
> 'The relationship is an evolving one, and much depends on developing mutual trust between doctor and patient.
>
> 'What the patient needs most during that first visit is an unhurried discussion of his or her symptoms, the diagnosis – if one can be made at that time – and the possible options for treatment.'
>
> – Dr. John Hassall, professor emeritus of rheumatology, Royal Prince Alfred Medical Centre, Sydney, Australia

Laboratory tests As we noted in Chapter 2, relatively few laboratory tests can actually help to diagnose the various types of arthritis. Instead, they are used mainly for ruling out other possible causes of joint pain, such as infections, side effects from drug treatment or cancer.

Getting the most from repeat appointments

Repeat appointments with the doctor are a hallmark of all chronic diseases, including arthritis. GPs have only a limited amount of time to spend with each patient at each appointment, so you can benefit by using that time wisely. Here are some practical tips for gaining the maximum benefit from your repeat appointment.

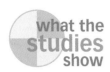

Prepare some talking points

Just as you did before your initial appointment, plan for your repeat appointment by thinking about the problems or questions that you have. Then write them down in the order of their urgency, so that you'll be sure that your most pressing issues will be dealt with. As a practical matter, try to limit yourself to three questions or concerns, since it's unlikely you'll have time to discuss more than that.

Remember why you are in the surgery

In a hit song from the 1960s, the singer announces that he 'just dropped in to see what condition my condition was in'. Before you decided to take charge of your arthritis, you may have approached your GP that way – with you sitting passively as the doctor asked you questions, felt your joints, and told you whether you were doing well or poorly. How you felt was not something you thought was worth mentioning – but it is the whole reason you are seeing your GP.

Office etiquette Adopting a take-charge approach during appointments will help you to get much more out of them. Telling your doctor how you're doing, how well the drug is working, whether the exercises are helping and how you are feeling will benefit you and will help your doctor to do the best for you. If you are having problems, you should say so and then spell out just what difficulties you are experiencing.

Many people have trouble taking this assertive approach with physicians, for fear of offending or insulting them. But actually, most doctors much prefer that patients provide them with that kind of feedback. Only by working together in this way can patient and doctor develop the treatment approach that will be the best possible one for the patient.

'Early on, I went to the doctor to see how I was doing ....Now I know that my doctor wanted me to tell him how I was doing, not the other way around.'

—Sharon Dorough, arthritis patient

Clear up uncertainties

Many doctors use jargon when discussing issues with patients, often blissfully unaware how incomprehensible it can be. Or they may simply fail to explain why they're recommending that you take a certain drug or stop taking another.

Whatever the reason, questions will almost inevitably arise during your visit – and what you don't understand could prevent you from gaining a better understanding of your arthritis. So don't be afraid to tell the doctor that you don't understand something or that you're confused. Most doctors won't mind going back over what they've said so that you can understand it.

Be a good reporter

When visiting the doctor, it's all too easy to make the 'forest-for-the-trees' mistake – perhaps becoming so distracted by a technical term you did not understand that you then failed to follow what the doctor was saying when discussing the possible side effects of a new drug that was being recommended.

Taking notes can help to ensure that important information doesn't get lost. It can also be very useful to bring along a friend or family member for backup: comparing notes with that person can help to fill in details that you might have missed.

Building your team

It has become increasingly apparent that a patient's interests may best be served by a 'treatment team'. In this team approach, the GP or rheumatologist (depending on the case) typically serves as doctor-in-charge, coordinating the care administered by other doctors or healthcare professionals. The team may include one or more of the following:

A nurse in a GP practice or hospital out-patient clinic can often provide information that the doctor missed, or clarify a comment the doctor made. A competent, caring nurse can answer questions about the side effects of a medication or get access to the doctor to provide an answer. Some nurses may have special experience in rheumatology and can help with advice on modifications in the home, office or even school to make your life a little easier. A nurse can become a counsellor, friend and advocate for you.

Physiotherapists prescribe exercises aimed at relieving pain and restoring lost muscle and joint function. In many cases, they can help you to restore the mobility you may have lost. They can work with you to create a personalized plan

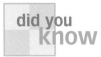
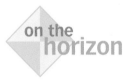
which consists of stretching as well as strength and aerobic exercises. They sometimes recommend water therapy, relaxation techniques, even biofeedback. Generally, a course of physiotherapy lasts just a few weeks, although long-term therapy may sometimes be recommended.

Occupational therapists evaluate their patients' ability to perform physical tasks both inside and outside the home. With the occupational therapist's advice, you can learn new ways of doing old things – from housework to cooking a meal. They often make suggestions for modifying the home and work environment so that you can function more efficiently and with less pain. Occupational therapists can also design and fit any splints or other devices you might need to support or protect weakened joints.

Dietitians can also help you to overcome the daily pains and aggravations of living with arthritis. When you are diagnosed with arthritis, what you eat can have a significant effect on your pain and health. A dietitian can explain the way in which foods interact, how the drugs you might be taking could deplete certain nutrients, and how vitamins might help. And, of course, proper nutrition will help you to lose weight if that is a problem – an often difficult task but one that for many patients is essential for reducing pain.

Orthopaedic surgeons are doctors who perform surgery on joints, including arthroscopy and joint-replacement surgery. GPs or rheumatologists may refer a patient with arthritis to an orthopaedic surgeon if drugs fail to relieve pain or disability.

Rehabilitation medicine specialists are general physicians whose specialized work involves prescribing special exercise programmes, crutches or devices that protect the joints.

Psychiatrists, psychologists and social workers can help patients with arthritis to cope with depression, anxiety, and other psychological problems often associated with having a chronic disease.

Family and friends are also vital resources in achieving your goals. Because arthritis is a long-term battle, you will occasionally need day-to-day help. When it is tough to get out of bed because your knees feel like hardened cement, you may sometimes need a friend or family member to provide a gentle shove towards that hot bath or shower. When you think about it, your family and friends have a vested interest in helping you to take charge of your condition.

When surgery is recommended: ask these questions

- What surgery are you recommending?

- Please describe what happens during the surgery.

- Exactly how will I be better off as a result of this surgery?

- What is the normal range of outcomes from this type of surgery?

- Please describe all the side effects of this surgery.

- How long will I be in hospital?

- How much pain will I experience, and what can be done to relieve it?

- Should I arrange to have someone to help me when I return home? And is there a self-help group near me?

- Will the surgery affect my ability to work?

- In which hospital will the surgery be performed? Does it have good surgical results?

- Do you have any printed information describing the surgery? And is there a web site I can access?

- Do you have any patients who underwent the same surgery that I can talk to?

- Can the surgery significantly affect or cure my osteoarthritis?

- Could the surgery make my condition worse than it is now?

If you think you might benefit from a team approach, don't hesitate to discuss the matter with your physician. Even better, suggest the specialist you have in mind – a physiotherapist, for example – and ask if your doctor could recommend a particular individual.

Too many cooks may indeed spoil the broth, but having the right number of specialists working for you can help to push you towards your goal of taking charge of your arthritis.

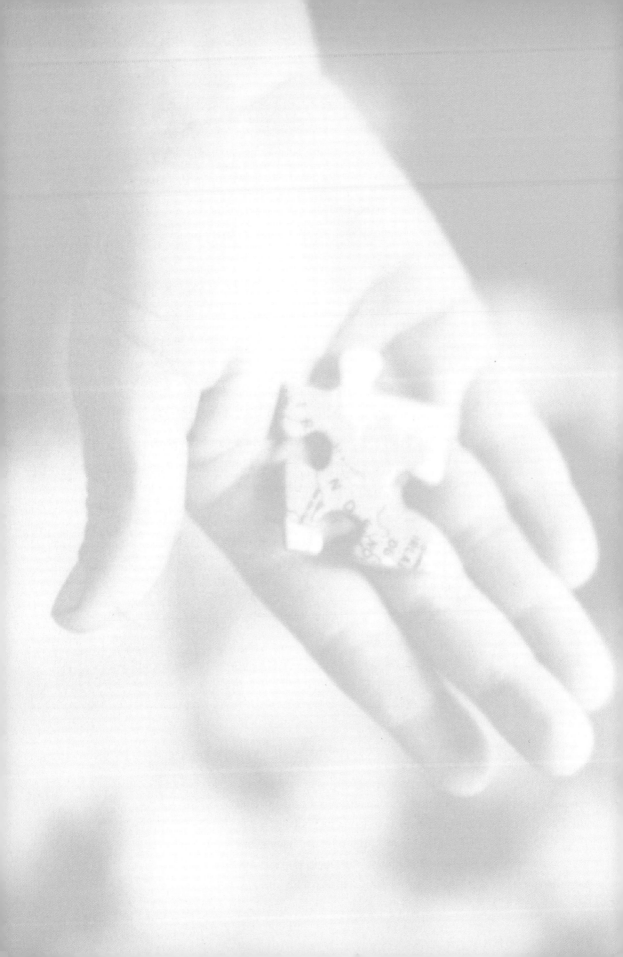

5

Drugs and surgery

A wide range of drugs is available

to combat arthritis, and if the pain

fails to respond to medication, there

are surgical options. Choosing

the right treatment can mean the

difference between living fully and

being imprisoned by your condition.

Painkilling medications

All types of arthritis have two things in common – they affect the joints in some way, and they cause pain. So it's not really surprising that many of the drugs used to treat arthritis help to reduce that pain. They range from paracetamol tablets to anti-inflammatory drugs to heat-producing creams and ointments. There are also surgical procedures that may offer some relief.

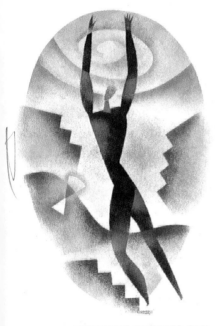

ARTHRITIS PATIENTS CAN CHOOSE from numerous drugs to relieve pain and stiffness. If one drug does not help, or causes unacceptable side effects, there is almost certainly another that will be worth trying.

The old and new

Drugs used to combat the pain of arthritis range from good old aspirin – used for more than a century – to several new and exciting drugs that have been available only since 1998. For the vast majority of arthritis patients who have osteoarthritis (OA), the drug news is mixed. Although many medications can help to relieve pain, no drug is yet available to do what OA patients need most: rebuild cartilage that has been damaged and lost over the years. (Here, however, certain dietary supplements may offer some help, as you'll see in Chapter 6.)

On the positive side, there are new drugs known as COX-2 inhibitors that are much less likely to cause stomach irritation and bleeding than older arthritis drugs. Some of the newest and most promising medications are reserved for people with rheumatoid arthritis and other forms of inflammatory arthritis.

> **◐ FACT** Your doctor may need to monitor the effects of your arthritis medication. A blood count, urinalysis or a liver function test may be required, depending on the drug used and its effect on you.

Which medicine?

There is a huge choice of drugs available for people with arthritis, partly because individuals respond in different ways to different drugs. There are currently some 27 brands of non-steroidal anti-inflammatory drugs (NSAIDs) on the UK market, with more awaiting approval from the Medicines Control Agency (MCA) – offering a choice, which means that you have a good chance of finding a drug that will work for you.

But no matter which medication you turn to, you should always research it thoroughly first. Try to obtain the latest information on safe dosages and side effects before you try it.

You and your doctor should weigh up how much a particular medicine can help you against its potential adverse side effects. The dosage prescribed usually starts low, and is then increased to a level that either helps or causes unpleasant side effects. If side effects do occur, the dosage can usually be reduced or you

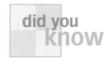

did you know

○ Fewer than one person in 20 has to stop a medicine because of side effects; aspirin is an exception, with one in six taken off the drug.

Know your drug – before you take it

Ask questions When taking a new medicine, ask about possible interactions with other drugs and if there are any special instructions relating to the absorption of the medicine. For example, is it important to take it between meals, with meals or just before you go to bed? Also, ask the doctor for the lowest possible dose of the drug that will still reduce your pain and inflammation. The lower the dose, the lower your chances of suffering serious side effects.

Side effects Since many arthritis drugs can cause anaemia, stomach ulcers and other gastrointestinal side effects, as well as kidney and liver damage, make sure your doctor orders the appropriate laboratory tests. Also, don't mistake an allergic reaction for an adverse reaction: allergic reactions usually result in hives or itching; adverse reactions are often more serious.

New medicines When you and your doctor decide that a new medicine is needed, your doctor should explain how the medicine is thought to work, what dose to take and the possible side effects. In addition, your doctor should ask you to return in one to two weeks for a safety check. You should report any unpleasant symptoms such as diarrhoea, abdominal pain, headaches, blurred vision or drowsiness.

can ask your doctor to try another drug. Make sure that you take your medications according to your GP's prescription, and that you notify your doctor about any complications or side effects. Never be tempted to borrow a medication from a friend who swears that it works wonders. It may not work as well for you and may even be dangerous.

Paracetamol – the first choice for pain relief

Sold under numerous brand names, paracetamol is usually effective for osteoarthritis patients who have mild to moderate joint pain. Paracetamol has been available since 1955 and is now the nation's leading pain reliever. The medication is not only effective but is also among the safest drugs that you can take. Considering the millions of doses consumed every year, it causes remarkably few side effects.

How it works Paracetamol relieves pain in a different way from NSAIDs. Aspirin, ibuprofen and other NSAIDs block the body's production of prostaglandins, the chemicals that increase inflammation and pain. However, paracetamol has no effect on prostaglandins; it works on the nervous system, raising the brain's threshold for pain.

Because paracetamol has no effect on prostaglandins, it does not relieve inflammation. So it won't be as effective as an NSAID against inflammatory types of arthritis. The benefit is that by leaving all the prostaglandins alone – including the 'good' ones that protect the stomach lining – paracetamol is far easier on the stomach than NSAIDs.

Gaining respect

Recent research has shown that many arthritis patients don't need NSAIDs after all. Although inflammation is certainly the main cause of the pain and joint damage in rheumatoid arthritis, scientists now know that inflammation is only rarely present in

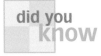

did you know

▷ Medicines sometimes stop working after months or years of providing pain relief. This is called tachyphylaxis. Although the reason why this happens may not be known, your doctor has two options: to increase the dose or prescribe a new medicine. Sometimes the failed medicine can be prescribed months or years later and will again be effective.

The problems of NSAIDs

Until a few years ago, doctors routinely prescribed NSAIDs rather than paracetamol for their arthritis patients. However, NSAIDs can cause serious adverse effects, particularly gastrointestinal problems.

The risks Within a year of starting treatment with an NSAID, up to 4 per cent of regular users develop stomach bleeding or painful ulcers. Prolonged use of NSAIDs also increases a patient's risk of developing liver disease and kidney disease (problems that are more likely to occur in people over 70) as well as high blood pressure.

On top of the risks comes the expense A prescription NSAID costs anywhere from £1.50 to £20 for 30 tablets; a supply of 32 paracetamol tablets costs about 75p, while 32 extra strength tablets (with codeine) costs under £2.

osteoarthritis, which is by far the most common form of the disease. When paracetamol was matched up against powerful NSAIDs in clinical studies involving osteoarthritis patients, the over-the-counter pain reliever proved surprisingly effective.

Help for painful knees One study, published in *The New England Journal of Medicine* in 1991, involved 184 patients with chronic, persistent knee pain as a result of osteoarthritis. Paracetamol was found to work as well as prescription-strength NSAIDs in relieving knee pain.

This and other studies have shown that paracetamol relieves mild to moderate osteoarthritis pain just as effectively as prescription NSAIDs – even in cases where the joints are actually inflamed. Because paracetamol was found to work as well as NSAIDs, but without the serious risks of regular NSAID use, it made sense that osteoarthritis patients should try paracetamol first.

Therefore whenever a patient presents with osteoarthritis of the knee and hip, doctors tend to prescribe paracetamol as a first choice, at an initial dose of up to 4000mg a day. If the patient shows no sign of improvement, the second choice tends to be the NSAID ibuprofen.

Paracetamol has more virtues than vices

Compared with the NSAID group of pain relievers, paracetamol is:

- Gentler on the gastrointestinal tract and much less likely to cause stomach bleeding or ulcers
- Not likely to raise blood pressure after prolonged use
- Less likely to cause liver or kidney disease
- Less likely to interact with other medications

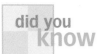
did you know

- In Continental Europe, suppositories are a popular way of administering NSAIDs because they reduce stomach pain and nausea. They are less popular in the UK because the British are more uncomfortable about taking drugs rectally.

Next drug, please

Paracetamol's gentleness on the stomach and gastrointestinal tract makes it the preferred first choice for easing the pain of osteoarthritis, which rarely involves inflammation (swelling, redness and warmth). But if you have tried paracetamol for a month and it fails to ease your pain, talk to your doctor about moving on to one of the NSAIDs.

Although NSAIDs do pose a greater risk of side effects, they may offer better pain relief than paracetamol. You may also find that combining paracetamol with an NSAID allows you to obtain pain relief with a lower (and safer) dose of NSAID than you would otherwise need. However, always talk to your doctor to find out if it is safe for you to combine two different pain relievers and what the recommended dosages should be.

A word of caution

Though in many ways safer than NSAIDs, paracetamol has the potential to cause serious illness and even death. Regular users – those who take paracetamol every day over many years – face an increased risk of liver or kidney damage. And both regular and casual users of paracetamol can experience serious liver damage if they take high amounts of the drug while also consuming three or more alcoholic drinks a day.

> **FACT** Taking paracetamol with food and avoiding alcohol can reduce the risk of kidney damage.

Watch the dosage Problems with paracetamol almost always result from doses far in excess of the maximum recommended dose of 4,000mg a day. (But for older people and anyone with pre-existing liver disease, even a modest overdose can be dangerous.) Make sure you keep track of how many tablets you have taken each day. Try counting out the tablets once a day so that you know not to take more than that amount. If pain is driving you to take more tablets, you should consult your doctor.

One other caution – it may be dangerous to take paracetamol if you have been fasting. A 1994 study in the *Journal of the American Medical Association* found that when people who have been fasting or who haven't been eating due to influenza or a stomach virus consume 'moderate overdoses' of paracetamol – between 4,000mg (the maximum recommended dose) and 10,000mg a day – they increase their risk of liver damage.

NSAIDs: relief from pain and inflammation

Non-steroidal anti-inflammatory drugs, or NSAIDs, are effective for arthritis patients who suffer from pain, inflammation or both – particularly those with inflammatory types of arthritis such as rheumatoid arthritis and ankylosing spondylitis.

First-line drugs If you are taking a drug for arthritis pain, you may well be taking one of the many NSAIDs that are on the market. ('Non-steroidal' means that these drugs do not include prednisolone or other members of the corticosteroid family of drugs, which are also anti-inflammatory.) NSAIDs are used against arthritis pain and many other types of pain, including headaches, menstrual pain and dental pain.

Aspirin, first marketed in1900, is now classified as an NSAID and all the NSAIDs have one thing in common; they relieve pain when taken in low doses, and pain

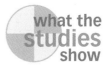

what the studies show

▷ According to a study in the April 2000 issue of the US *Journal of Rheumatology,* most patients who take both paracetamol and an NSAID for osteoarthritis say that the NSAID is more helpful against pain. But paracetamol was better tolerated; 33 per cent of the patients continued taking paracetamol for more than two years, versus only 21 per cent for ibuprofen, 17 per cent for naproxen, and 19 per cent for diclofenac.

caution

Patients with a history of asthma attacks, hives or other allergic reactions to aspirin should avoid NSAIDs.

How to take NSAIDs – and keep your stomach happy

Gastrointestinal irritation is by far the most common (and often the most serious) problem posed by NSAIDs. However, if you take an NSAID for your arthritis, there are several precautions you can take to make sure you don't upset your stomach:

1 Take the drug with a glass of water and during meals.

2 Don't lie down immediately after taking the drug; wait at least 15 to 30 minutes.

3 Limit your alcohol intake to three drinks a day or less, since combining NSAIDs with heavy drinking increases the likelihood of gastrointestinal irritation.

4 Ask your doctor about instituting a drug holiday. Taking NSAIDs a few days on and a few days off can give the stomach some time to heal itself. If the pain and inflammation become too intense, paracetamol may be an alternative during the off days.

5 Consult your doctor before mixing different types of NSAIDs, even if you intend to take both drugs in low doses. Combining NSAIDs – especially in anti-inflammatory doses – can greatly increase the risk of stomach irritation.

6 If you take occasional doses of aspirin, products that contain antacids – such as 'buffered' aspirin brands – may reduce stomach irritation, although they may not be gentler to the stomach with prolonged use. Enteric-coated aspirin may also help.

The special coating prevents aspirin from dissolving in the stomach; instead it dissolves in the small intestine. However, a disadvantage of this particular form of NSAID is that because of the coating you will have to wait longer before feeling any pain relief.

and inflammation when taken at high dosages. Many people with osteoarthritis take NSAIDs for pain relief – but most of them don't need high doses, since inflammation often isn't present in OA. But for people with OA who also suffer with inflammation or for those who have any type of inflammatory arthritis, taking a high-dose NSAID to reduce inflammation can be extremely helpful, since the inflammation damages the joints and causes much of the pain.

There are many NSAIDs available over the counter, such as ibruprofen, among others. They are available under numerous brand names, some of which are higher-dose, prescription-only formulations.

The pros and cons of NSAIDs

NSAIDs work by preventing the body from producing pain-inducing chemicals called prostaglandins. They shut off the 'bad' prostaglandins by blocking an enzyme called cyclooxygenase (COX) 2.

Double-edged swords But, unfortunately, in addition to blocking COX-2, standard NSAIDs also block the COX-1 enzyme, which produces 'good' prostaglandins that protect the lining of the stomach and other parts of the gastrointestinal tract by regenerating their mucus lining. Without this mucus lining, the gastrointestinal tract can be damaged by acidic and caustic digestive fluids that are always present. Not surprisingly, NSAIDs in prescription-strength doses are more likely to cause problems than nonprescription NSAIDs.

> ● FACT If you are at risk of developing gastrointestinal complications, perhaps you should try diclofenac sodium (Arthrotec). It combines the NSAID diclofenac with misoprostol, man-made prostaglandins that help to protect the gastrointestinal tract.

While NSAIDs help to relieve pain and inflammation, they can also cause major gastrointestinal problems, including ulcers and significant bleeding. Every year in the UK, 1 to 2 per cent of all patients taking NSAIDs are hospitalized as a result of severe gastrointestinal problems and around 2,500–3,000 deaths are attributed to the drugs.

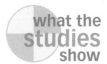

what the **studies** show

● From 40 to 60 per cent of people who use either prescription or non-prescription NSAIDs over long periods of time develop shallow injuries ('erosions') in the lining of their stomachs or small intestines. Between 10 and 30 per cent of long-term users will end up with deeper injuries, such as ulcers.

But these statistics should be kept in perspective: NSAIDs are one of the most popular classes of drugs and most of the people who use them don't experience any serious complications.

Choosing the right NSAID

All NSAIDs work in basically the same way, so you might expect that patients would benefit from whichever NSAID they took. But in reality the way arthritis patients respond to an NSAID is individual: quite often, patients who notice no improvement from one NSAID will do quite well when switched to another.

Sometimes patients must try several different NSAIDs before finding the right one: a drug that is both effective and does not cause side effects. As a general rule, if an NSAID is going to work for you, it will be effective within seven to 14 days.

COX-2 inhibitors – a kinder, gentler type of NSAID

The latest weapon in the pharmaceutical arsenal against arthritis pain is a new class of NSAID known as COX-2 inhibitors. Compared with the standard NSAID drugs, these new prescription medications are less likely to cause bleeding and other gastrointestinal problems.

That's good news for the estimated 30 per cent of NSAID users who experience persistent gastrointestinal symptoms from using the older drugs and the 10 per cent of users who are forced to discontinue taking NSAIDs because of unpleasant side effects.

A new role for an old standby

Aspirin remains a useful drug for occasional arthritis pain, but it has largely been replaced by newer NSAIDs in treating rheumatoid arthritis and other inflammatory types of the disease. This is because aspirin causes greater irritation to the stomach lining and is less convenient to take (an anti-inflammatory dose of aspirin requires taking four to six doses a day compared with only one or two daily doses of many other NSAIDs).

But although its role in treating arthritis is fading, aspirin remains extremely useful for other purposes:

● It can significantly reduce the risk of heart attack and stroke, probably by reducing clot formation, when taken in low doses.

● Taking aspirin within 24 hours of a heart attack, and then daily for the next month, reduces the risk of dying from the heart attack by about 25 per cent.

● Aspirin may help to prevent memory loss in older people and slow down mental deterioration in people who are already senile.

● It may protect against colon cancer and may help in preventing other cancers as well.

How it works All NSAIDs relieve pain in the same basic way – by blocking an enzyme called cyclooxygenase, or COX. As discussed before, this enzyme produces prostaglandins, important chemicals that perform many different functions in the body.

As recently as 1991, researchers discovered that COX comes in two forms: the 'good' COX-1, which produces helpful prostaglandins to keep the gastrointestinal tract coated with protective mucus; and the 'bad' COX-2 that is responsible for producing prostaglandins that play a big part in causing pain and inflammation in the body.

caution

People who need a COX-2 inhibitor but are allergic to sulfa drugs should avoid Celebrex, which can cause similar allergic reactions. Vioxx and Mobic don't cause such reactions.

The standard NSAID takes a rough and ready approach to the COX enzymes: it eases pain and inflammation by blocking COX-2, but unfortunately it also blocks COX-1, leaving your gastrointestinal tract susceptible to irritation that can cause ulcers and bleeding. Here's where COX-2 inhibitors, NSAIDs designed to affect only the COX-2 enzyme, come in.

Sorting out the hype from reality

In 1996, Mobic (meloxicam) became the first COX-2 inhibitor to be licensed in the UK. Vioxx (rofecoxib) was approved in 1999 and Celebrex (celecoxib) in 2000. Additional COX-2 inhibitors are expected to become available in the near future. Although the COX-2 inhibitors represent a major advance in arthritis treatment, it is important to consider the following:

1 The many studies that have compared COX-2s with standard NSAIDs show that COX-2s are no more effective against pain and inflammation. If you are using a standard NSAID that works for you and is not causing any problems, switching to one of the COX-2s is not necessarily going to be better for you.

2 Although COX-2s cause fewer gastrointestinal side effects than standard NSAIDs, they are not risk-free. Clinical studies show that ulcers, irritation and other problems still occur with COX-2 inhibitors, although significantly less often than with standard NSAIDs.

3 COX-2 inhibitors are much more expensive than standard NSAIDs, which may be significant as GPs are increasingly encouraged to choose the most cost-effective drugs.

4 Unlike aspirin, COX-2s do not prevent the blood from clotting, so they are not helpful against heart attack and stroke. If you take COX-2s, don't stop taking aspirin if it has been prescribed for heart or stroke problems.

Are COX-2 inhibitors for you?

The following questions can help you to work out whether you may be a candidate for COX-2 therapy:

1 Do you have a previous or current history of ulcer disease?

did you know

The COX-2 inhibitors Celebrex and Vioxx are no safer than standard NSAIDs when it comes to impairing kidney function in healthy older people, according to a July 2000 study in the *Annals of Internal Medicine.*
If you're over 65 and regularly take Celebrex, Vioxx, or any other NSAID for arthritis, ask your doctor for a blood test to monitor your kidney function.

2 Have you stopped using standard NSAIDs because you weren't able to tolerate them?

3 Are you older than 65? (Older people face an increased risk of bleeding and other gastrointestinal problems caused by standard NSAIDs.)

4 Are you currently taking a corticosteroid? (People taking prednisolone or other corticosteroids are at increased risk of gastrointestinal bleeding.)

If yes, to one or more of the above, COX-2 therapy may be for you.

Different NSAIDs, different risks

In the UK, 1 to 2 per cent of all patients taking NSAIDs are hospitalized because of the adverse gastrointestinal effects of the drugs. It has also been estimated that between 2,500 and 3,000 deaths every year can be attributed to the use of these drugs. Nevertheless, the use of NSAIDs is growing and it could be said that the more enthusiastic users are putting themselves at risk. Studies have shown that some NSAIDs are more likely than others to cause serious problems.

Slight risk

Celecoxib (Celebrex)
Todolac (Lodine)
Ibuprofen (Motrin)
Meloxicam (Mobic)
Nabumetone (Relifex)
Rofecoxib (Vioxx)

Serious risk

Acetylsalicylic acid (Aspirin)*
Diflunisal (Dolobid)
Fenbufen (Lederfen)
Indometacin (Indocid)
Meclofenamate (Meclomen)
Piroxicam (Feldene)

Moderate risk

Diclofenac (Voltarol)
Ketoprofen (Orudis)
Naproxen (Naprosyn)

*More than three 325mg tablets daily

Mobic's COX-2 status queried in the USA

In the USA, the Food and Drug Administration (FDA) approved Mobic as an NSAID in 2000 but argued against classifying it as a COX-2 inhibitor because it claimed that Mobic selectively inhibits COX-2 at therapeutic doses. As required by the FDA, drugs labelled as COX-2 inhibitors must target COX-2 exclusively – even at twice their therapeutic dose – and Mobic does not meet that standard.

In the UK, Mobic was licensed as a COX-2 inhibitor in 1996. Comparison studies have apparently shown that it causes few side effects than standard NSAIDs.

Could visco-supplementation help to soothe sore knees?

If you have osteoarthritis of the knee and have not been helped by paracetamol or NSAIDs, you may want to consider a new procedure called visco-supplementation. It uses hyaluronic acid, a natural component of synovial fluid that helps to lubricate the knee and other joints.

In 1998, the MCA licensed the first visco-supplementation medication for use in patients with knee pain caused by osteoarthritis. The substance, Hyalgan, is administered by five injections, a week apart. The doctor numbs your skin and injects the jelly-like hyaluronic acid directly into the knee.

How it works Once in the joint, it replaces the body's own hyaluronic acid that is lost when a joint is affected by osteoarthritis. Researchers have suggested several possible mechanisms to explain how visco-supplementation may help to relieve knee pain. One theory is that it bolsters the joint's shock-absorbing ability, so cushioning and lessening the pain of movement. Recent studies show that pain relief from visco-supplementation can last as long as nine to 12 months and that the injections can be safely repeated.

● FACT A course of visco-supplementation costs around £180, although it is available on the NHS. It is also available through some private health insurance schemes.

Visco-supplementation can undoubtedly help some patients, but rheumatologists seem to be taking a wait-and-see attitude toward the treatment. It may be especially useful for patients with osteoarthritis of the knee who are not helped by NSAIDs or who cannot tolerate the drugs.

Side effects They are usually mild and include increased pain and swelling of the knee, as well as a rash, itching or both at the injection site.

Corticosteroids offer relief – at a price

The introduction of prednisolone (a well-known cortisone derivative) in the 1950s revolutionized the treatment of rheumatoid arthritis (RA). After patients took oral prednisolone for a few days, they found that their inflammation was controlled and their mobility restored.

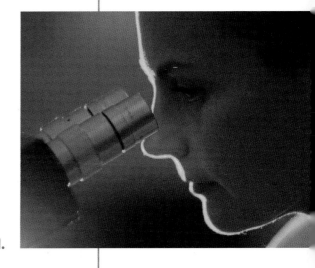

It did not take long to discover the dark side of corticosteroids: the initial dose has to be increased to maintain the benefits. This can lead to serious side effects. Corticosteroids still remain one of the most effective of all treatments for patients with severe rheumatoid arthritis, although physicians try to use them as a last resort.

How they work Steroids vary in their action; some act for longer, but have slower onset of pain relief, while others act faster with a quicker onset of relief. Steroids seem to prevent the release of certain chemicals that tend to inflame and degrade cartilage and its

caution

Steroids should never be taken orally by patients as a treatment for osteoarthritis, although they can be injected safely into the knee joint.

Targeting the joint

By injecting steroids directly into a painful joint, rheumatologists are able to reduce the risk of serious complications that can occur when steroids are administered by mouth or by injection into muscles.

Minimizing infection Anyone considering corticosteroid injections should weigh their temporary benefits against possible risks, particularly the risk of infecting the joint, which can be a serious matter. To minimize the risk of infection, physicians generally will not administer a steroid injection if the patient has an infection elsewhere in the body, such as a urinary or respiratory infection, for example.

supporting structures in the joint. New evidence suggests that corticosteroids also block cytokines, another class of chemicals responsible for inflammation.

> **⊙ FACT** You should never abruptly stop taking corticosteroids. This can lead to a flare-up of symptoms. Instead you should be weaned from them gradually. Your doctor will be able to help you with this.

A dramatic improvement As treatments for rheumatoid arthritis, corticosteroids are either taken by mouth or injected by a doctor. In either case, they must be carefully administered, typically in 'microdose' therapy: low-dose therapy that relieves inflammation while avoiding the serious side effects that higher doses can cause. In severe cases, steroids can improve the disease dramatically, often producing a sense of well-being in the patient. But, eventually, the drug stops working and side effects can occur.

A point about precautions

Serious side effects don't usually occur when corticosteroids are taken for only one or two months. Even in people who require large doses, many of the side effects will disappear after the medicine is stopped. However, you should be aware of them:

- Fluid retention. A person can gain 10lb to 20lb, causing high blood pressure.

- Bone loss. Steroids can cause loss of calcium from the bones, which can lead to osteoporosis and fractures of the back or other bones.

- Other side effects include cataracts; easy bruising of the skin; emotional changes; risk of infection; destruction of large joints, such as the hips; stunted growth in children.

Declaring war on rheumatoid arthritis with DMARDs

The NSAIDs have long been the mainstay of rheumatoid arthritis treatment, and for good reason: they are very effective in suppressing inflammation, the destructive force that can lead to severe pain and joint damage. But in the past few years, the treatment of rheumatoid arthritis has expanded to include a new class of drug, known as disease-modifying anti-rheumatic drugs, or DMARDs.

Move over NSAIDs The NSAIDs remain important in RA therapy but rheumatologists no longer rely on them as heavily, for several reasons.

- The high NSAID doses needed to relieve inflammation can sometimes cause serious complications.

- Experts realized that people often experienced worsening joint damage, despite using pain-relieving NSAIDs.

- The DMARDs offer certain advantages over NSAIDs. DMARDs not only reduce inflammation but also slow down the joint destruction that, with NSAIDs, can continue even when inflammation has been quelled.

did you know

- To bring about prompt pain relief, rheumatologists often inject corticosteroids directly into sore joints of patients with arthritis. But repeated corticosteroid injections may damage cartilage, especially in weight-bearing joints such as the hip and knee. For this reason, injections into the same joint should usually be spaced at least four months apart.

Once used only when other treatments had failed or only when joint damage became apparent, DMARDs are potent drugs that can have serious side effects.

But in a major shift in the way rheumatoid arthritis is treated, many physicians now prescribe DMARDs as soon as the condition is diagnosed, in an aggressive effort to halt the disease's progression and to prevent the damage it can cause to joints and internal organs.

The older DMARDS – are they still as effective?

Methotrexate

Although it has been used for decades to treat cancer and severe psoriasis, methotrexate was licensed for treating rheumatoid arthritis only in 2002.

Its potential was discovered when dermatologists prescribed it for psoriasis patients who also had rheumatoid arthritis, and noticed that their arthritis greatly improved. Use of methotrexate as a treatment for rheumatoid arthritis is steadily increasing and in the UK and the USA, it now ranks as one of the most commonly prescribed DMARDs.

How it works Rheumatoid arthritis occurs when the immune system begins to attack the body's own joints, causing the chronic inflammation that can eventually destroy cartilage and bone. Like many DMARDs, methotrexate is an immuno-suppressant, which means that it blunts the immune system's assault on the joints, thereby reducing the destructive and painful inflammation that is associated with the condition.

Methotrexate is not only extremely effective for many rheumatoid arthritis patients, but also works faster than many other DMARDs, with improvement sometimes noticed within two weeks. It also has a good safety record; fewer than 5 per cent of patients have to stop using it because of side effects. Methotrexate is usually given orally, once a week.

Side effects Since methotrexate can cause liver damage, patients need regular liver-function tests to check for potential damage and must not drink alcohol heavily while taking the drug. Pregnant women

caution

Since methotrexate can sometimes damage the liver, patients taking it should receive regular liver function tests – blood tests that can detect liver damage before it becomes severe.

should never take methotrexate because it may cause serious birth defects or even kill the foetus. Methotrexate may also deplete sperm counts in men.

> **● FACT** Methotrexate can lower your absorption of folic acid, causing a deficiency of this important vitamin. Therefore some doctors recommend that their patients take a small daily supplement containing folic acid to prevent this potential shortfall.

Gold

Since the 1920s, gold therapy has been an important treatment for rheumatoid arthritis and remained a common option until methotrexate emerged in the USA in the 1980s. It can be administered either orally (given daily for an indefinite period of time) or by injection. The usual way is to inject it into the muscle weekly for four or five months. Maintenance injections are then given every two to four weeks indefinitely.

Oral gold (Ridaura) is easier to take and causes fewer side effects, but injectable gold is usually more effective. Some doctors begin with oral gold and, if no improvement is apparent, move on to injectable gold for six months.

How it works Gold is slow-acting but helps to suppress joint inflammation, although experts are uncertain how it accomplishes this. Gold must be used for several months before improvement occurs. After using gold for two to four months, patients may notice reduced morning stiffness; joint inflammation, along with pain and tenderness, may start to diminish after four to six months.

Side effects About 10 per cent of children and adults on gold experience anaemia, low white-blood-cell count, or liver-function test abnormalities. Gold can also harm the kidneys and cause a skin rash that disappears when the dosage is reduced.

Sulfasalazine

Developed in the 1930s, this drug was not widely used, but impressive results from recent studies have sparked renewed interest. The drug works well for many rheumatoid arthritis patients while rarely causing serious side effects. It seems to be quite effective when taken in combination with methotrexate.

did you know

● Patients with moderate to severe rheumatoid arthritis, and who can't tolerate or haven't responded to DMARD therapy, may be interested in the Prosorba column procedure (the treatment is available in the USA but not yet in Britain). A coffee-mug-sized device apparently filters out antibodies and immune complexes that damage the joints. Patients undergo 12 weekly outpatient sessions, each lasting about 2 hours.

How it works Experts still don't know just how sulfasalazine works. It seems to suppress the inflammatory activity of rheumatoid arthritis. It is licensed in the UK and widely used here for RA and in Europe, both for pain relief and arthritis. Though it has not yet been approved in the USA, many US rheumatologists prescribe it, when other drugs have proven unsuccessful.

Side effects The most common are nausea, headaches, dizziness, allergic reactions, such as rashes, and gastrointestinal upset. In rare cases, the drug can produce serious blood and liver toxicity.

Hydroxychloroquine

Long used as a treatment for malaria, hydroxychloroquine (its brand name is Plaquenil) became a rheumatoid arthritis drug when malaria patients with the condition noticed that it improved their arthritis. Hydroxychloroquine helps to relieve pain in many people with rheumatoid arthritis, but arthritis experts differ in their opinion of it: some recommend its use only after other drugs have failed, while others regard it as an effective drug that seldom causes side effects. It takes many months of treatment to show any benefit.

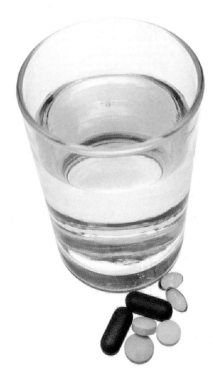

How it works The medication is taken orally and almost always in combination with other drugs. Although experts are not sure exactly how it works, it can dramatically help some patients. Taking hydroxychloroquine, may also mean that the amount of corticosteroid needed to help to relieve pain and inflammation can be reduced.

Side effects They include nausea, skin rashes, the presence of blood or protein in the urine, abnormal liver function and injury to the back of the eye. Patients should undergo an eye examination every three to six months.

Penicillamine

A synthetic offspring of penicillin, penicillamine is most effective for two kinds of arthritis patients — those with the specific genetic marker HLA-DR2 and those unresponsive to other DMARDs. Always taken with an NSAID or sometimes a steroid, penicillamine is considered a medication of last resort, yet some people with arthritis respond only to penicillamine.

How it works Its effectiveness as an arthritis drug was discovered by accident. Penicillamine binds to heavy metals such as gold and removes them from the body in patients. When it was used to treat gold overdosage in patients with RA, it relieved the arthritis. Penicillamine seems to act on the immune system in unknown ways to suppress the condition.

Side effects Mild side effects include loss of taste, as well as blood in the urine and abnormal liver function. On rare occasions, a muscular condition called myasthenia gravis can occur, causing a weakness of muscles. Patients should undergo regular blood and urine tests while taking the medication.

The newest DMARDS

Etanercept

Revolutionary but extremely expensive, this new-generation DMARD was licensed in the UK in 2000. Etanercept is used to treat moderate to severe rheumatoid arthritis and is taken twice weekly by injection. Clinical trials have shown the drug (brand name Enbrel) to be both well tolerated and effective, decreasing pain and morning stiffness and reducing joint swelling and tenderness. It won the Prix Galien, the top UK award for drug innovation in 2002.

How it works Etanercept is a 'designer drug' specifically created to reduce levels of tumour necrosis factor (TNF), a protein produced by the immune system that seems to play a major role in causing both inflammation and joint damage in rheumatoid arthritis. (TNF has also been implicated in other chronic health problems, including inflammatory bowel disease and congestive heart failure.) Etanercept takes aim at TNF-alpha, the most notorious form of the protein.

In small doses, TNF plays a useful function in the body's immune response by helping cells repair themselves. But in rheumatoid arthritis and some other immune disorders, too much TNF is produced and it ends up destroying healthy tissue such as heart muscle (in congestive heart failure) and cartilage and bone (in rheumatoid arthritis).

what the studies show

A study reported in the August 1997 issue of *The Lancet*, showed that 72 per cent of patients who were given a corticosteroid (prednisolone), methotrexate and sulfasalazine together showed improvement in their rheumatoid arthritis compared with improvement in only 49 per cent of the control group.

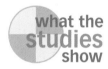

what the studies show

▶ Multiple doses of infliximab combined with methotrexate can achieve long-term control of rheumatoid arthritis, according to a study in the April 2000 issue of the US *Journal of Rheumatology*. In a study carried out on patients at three medical centres, the combination therapy halted progression of the disease for up to 40 weeks. Most patients showed significant improvement after one or two weeks of treatment.

In order to damage a cell, TNF must first latch onto 'docking molecules' on the surface of the cell, called TNF receptors. Etanercept essentially consists of millions of man-made TNF receptors. When etanercept is injected into the bloodstream, these TNF receptors mop up the TNF alpha in the bloodstream, which prevents the protein from docking onto cells and causing an inflammatory response.

Help where most needed Etanercept is seen as a major breakthrough in the treatment of rheumatoid arthritis because it helps most patients who have failed to benefit from any other therapies. It has also been found effective when used in children suffering from the juvenile form of the disease.

Although etanercept is injected, it can be administered at home and is sold in prefilled syringes. (The drug must be kept refrigerated because it is a natural protein that can break down at room temperature.) At a yearly cost of about £9,300, etanercept is currently the most expensive of all treatments for rheumatoid arthritis.

Side effects Some patients report mild reactions at the injection site and upper respiratory tract infections.

Infliximab

Licensed as a treatment for rheumatoid arthritis in 1999, this designer drug also knocks out tumour necrosis factor, but it works in a different way to etanercept. Infliximab (its brand name is Remicade) consists of millions of identical antibodies, known as monoclonal antibodies, that have been synthesized specifically to target TNF-alpha. Like etanercept, infliximab can produce a dramatic improvement in rheumatoid arthritis patients who haven't responded to other therapies.

How it works Just as the body's natural antibodies home in on and destroy bacteria and viruses, infliximab's antibodies latch onto and inactivate TNF-alpha. This greatly reduces the amount of TNF-alpha available to inflame and damage the joints.

Infliximab is administered intravenously by a healthcare professional, a procedure that takes about 2 hours and is given at four-week or eight-week intervals. A year of treatment with infliximab costs about £8,500.

The oral tradition

If you don't like injections, you'll like the DMARD leflunomide (Arava), which can be taken orally, usually in 10mg, 20mg or 100mg tablets. In fact, it is typically prescribed in a 'loading dose' of 100mg a day for the first three days, then 20mg daily afterwards. (Patients who suffer side effects may have their dose lowered to 10mg a day.)

How it works Rather than focusing on TNF-alpha, like the newest DMARDs etanercept and infliximab, leflunomide works by disabling lymphocytes, white blood cells that play a role in the immune system's attack on the joints. It does the job by neutralizing an enzyme in the white cells. Studies show that leflunomide is at least as effective as methotrexate in slowing the progression of joint damage in rheumatoid arthritis patients. Equally promising, 40 to 60 per cent of patients respond to this drug.

Side effects Because leflunomide is fairly new, no data exists on the potential long-term side effects. Your doctor should perform frequent tests, at least in the beginning of treatment, to monitor its effects on your body.

Surgical options

Before the 1960s there wasn't much that surgery could do for osteoarthritis. Then, it was common to smooth out irregular joint surfaces or fuse a joint, helping the pain but causing other problems; imagine trying to walk with a locked knee.

New joints and more By far the greatest surgical advance in arthritis treatment is total replacement of an arthritic joint, a procedure known as total arthroplasty. Numerous joints can now

continued on page 160

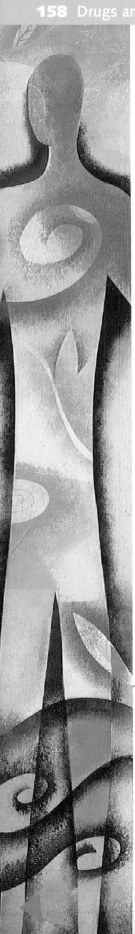

Winning the drug wars

Forty-seven-year-old Gill Boreham from Cornwall has had her fair share of drugs to help her to cope with arthritis and, until fairly recently, had to endure some nasty side effects.

Arthritis ran in Gill's family: her mother had rheumatoid arthritis and her father developed osteoarthritis. When she was a teenager Gill suffered problems with the lower part of her back. Gill says that as a child someone took away the chair she was about to sit on; she landed badly and that was the start of her problems.

Gill coped with her backaches coming and going until her mid 30s when, after the birth of her third child, she developed more nagging pains in her lower back.

'I was a very fit person and enjoyed aerobics and cycling,' says Gill. 'I was very active with my children and just put the back pain down to wear and tear taken by a mum with a busy family life. It wasn't until I went to aerobics and found it difficult to walk the next day, and then found myself not being able to get off my bike at the end of the day, during a cycling holiday, that I realized I needed to visit the doctor.'

Gill was told by her GP that she had probably pulled a muscle and she was prescribed a nonsteroidal anti-inflammatory drug or NSAID. However, the pain kept coming back, she says.

Gill's GP decided to refer her for X-rays, but these revealed that there was no disc damage to her back. This wasn't the news she was expecting.

'I felt totally shattered' says Gill, 'I could not believe I could be in so much pain, yet the discs in my back were not affected.' More anti-inflammatories were prescribed and Gill was referred to a rheumatologist.

The rheumatologist took one look at the X-rays and could immediately see the problem. Gill, at the age of 37, and with her son only six years old, had ankylosing spondylitis (AS). This can be a challenging disease to diagnose and often escapes detection in women as it is much more common in men.

It took a while for Gill to come to terms with the diagnosis. 'If I was aged 60 or 70, I could have perhaps understood it, but being as young as I was, I just didn't want to accept it,' says Gill. 'I thought I could carry on as if nothing had changed.'

When the pain spread to her shoulders, neck, hips and feet, even stronger anti-inflammatories

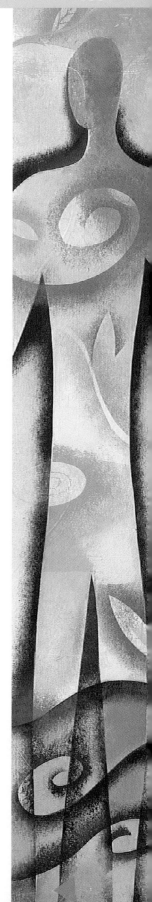

were prescribed for her and after suffering terrible pains in her sternum, Gill went back to the rheumatologist.

The specialist prescribed the NSAID Lodine. Gill took this drug for a few years without experiencing any side effects, but after a bout of severe back pain Gill was given Brexidol, another form of NSAID, to try.

Gill's GP also recommended that she should attend Arthritis Care's 'Challenging Arthritis' course. The course helped her enormously.

'It really helped me come to terms with things and to start realizing that I needed help and that it was all right to ask for it. I found it difficult coping with the fatigue, which is such a huge problem with AS. But the course gave me pointers as to how I could cope best with it.'

However, having come to terms with her condition in her own mind, three months after taking the latest medication, Gill had another setback. 'I began to suffer stomach problems,' she says. 'If I ate fat or acidic fresh fruit like oranges I would start to feel very poorly.'

Her GP performed tests and diagnosed a duodenal ulcer.

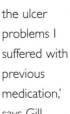

'Arthritis Care's course really helped me come to terms with things' says Gill.

Gill was given another drug, Celebrex, which is a new class of NSAID known as a COX-2 inhibitor. Compared with some of the other standard drugs used for arthritis pain, it is far less likely to cause bleeding and other gastrointestinal problems.

'For the past 18 months now I have been taking Celebrex and although it may not at times keep my pain at bay as much as I would like, at least I don't have the ulcer problems I suffered with previous medication,' says Gill.

'My life has changed a lot. Although I had to give up full-time work, I now lead self-management courses for Arthritis Care. To be able to share my experience with others and to help them feel they have the knowledge to break the pain cycle makes things seem worth while.'

Celebrex was licensed for use in the UK in 2000 and COX-2 inhibitors represent a major advance in the treatment of arthritis. Of course, they are not suitable for everyone and you should always seek medical advice before taking it.

be replaced with artificial ones, including the shoulders, elbows, wrists, fingers, ankles and even the toes. But the most common – and the most successful – joint replacement operations involve the hip and the knee.

Each year in the UK, some 44,000 hip-replacement and more than 35,000 knee-replacement operations are performed. The procedures relieve arthritis symptoms in knees and hips about 95 per cent of the time – a much higher success rate than for any other commonly performed operation for arthritis. On the following pages, you'll find a list of surgical options that are available.

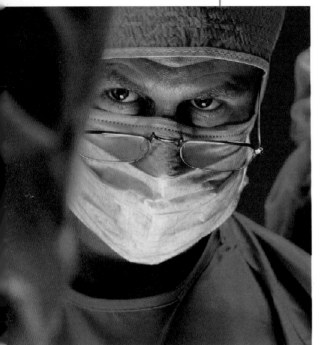

Is surgery for you?

There are six key questions that you should ask yourself to determine if you are a candidate for undergoing a surgical procedure:

1 Has your pain interfered with too many enjoyable things in your life?

2 Do you require strong painkillers?

3 Have you tried all other options to cope with the pain?

4 Are your goals realistic?

5 Are you as physically fit as you can be for activities?

6 Have you been able to discuss the risks of surgery with a health professional?

If, after a great deal of thought, you decide to have surgery, your GP will be able to refer you to the relevant orthopaedic surgeon at your nearest hospital. An orthopaedic surgeon is a medical doctor with extensive training in diagnosing and surgically treating the musculoskeletal system, including bones, joints, ligaments, tendons, muscles and nerves. If you decide to opt for private treatment, you should bear the following in mind:

❯ Your GP may still be able to give you a referral but you may also want to do your own homework and find the very best specialist in your area.

❯ *The Good Doctor Guide* by Catherine Vassallo (Simon & Schuster, 1997) may be helpful.

If you are claiming treatment as part of a medical insurance policy, your choice of doctor may be determined by the insurance company who will request operations are carried out by specific surgeons at specific hospitals.

Replacing joints: the techniques keep improving

For people with joints severely damaged by osteoarthritis or rheumatoid arthritis, total joint-replacement surgery can be a godsend. The operation offers miraculous improvement for severely disabled people who would otherwise spend their lives bedridden or confined to a wheelchair.

The hip was the first joint to be replaced, in a procedure that was pioneered by UK surgeon Sir John Charnley in the 1960s. In this surgery, an entire joint is removed and replaced by an artificial joint made of durable plastic, metal or ceramic. Thanks to improvements through the years, total hip and knee replacement are now highly successful operations with a failure rate of only 1 or 2 per cent.

Now what? Patients typically return home four or five days after the surgery. Most are able to walk two to three months after hip surgery and about three months after knee replacement. (You need to be aware that knee surgery tends to cause more postoperative pain.) Full recovery from either hip or knee replacement surgery can take up to a year.

Surgical advances All artificial joints wear out eventually. Fortunately, with today's newer materials and improved surgical techniques, most joints can be expected to last for 20 years or more. Joints wear out faster in younger people, whose higher activity levels put more stress and strain on them.

Replacing an artificial joint (a procedure known as revision arthroplasty) isn't as effective as the original; there is more pain and less freedom of movement. In fact, the eventual need for the second operation is a common argument for delaying the original surgery for as long as possible.

On the other hand, the advice from some doctors – 'put off your joint replacement until you can't stand the pain' – seems at odds with the mission of a patient who wants to take charge of his or her arthritis. Today's hip and knee-replacement operations are almost always successful and consistently provide total or near-total relief from pain for many years.

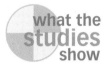

what the studies show

A study in the April 2000 issue of the US magazine *Bone and Joint Surgery* suggests that many people may not have to worry about undergoing a second hip-replacement operation. Researchers who followed up on hip replacements carried out between 1970 and 1972 found that 90 per cent of the 327 hips replaced were still functioning until the patient died or 25 years later for patients who were still alive. Today's hip replacements should last even longer, since they use a 'cementless' technique that provides a firmer fit.

Having confidence in your operation

If you decide to go ahead, here are some questions that you might like to ask or research before you undergo a joint-replacement operation:

- ◐ What is the success rate for this surgery?

- ◐ Are there any potential complications?

- ◐ How will I feel after the operation and what do I need to know about aftercare?

- ◐ How much time am I likely to need to recover from the operation?

- ◐ How many years has the surgeon been in practice?

- ◐ Will the surgeon be performing the joint procedure alone? If not, who will be assisting with the operation?

- ◐ Will the surgeon be in the operating theatre the entire time?

- ◐ What is the MRSA infection rate in the hospital where you will have the operation? What procedures are in place there for handling infection?

Other options

If drugs or other nonsurgical treatments aren't helping you – but you don't yet need to replace a joint – you may find relief from several limited types of surgery.

Arthroscopy This minimally invasive procedure, also known as 'keyhole' surgery, involves operating through small incisions in the skin. In arthritis treatment, arthroscopy is used mainly on knees. It can be quite effective in easing pain and stiffness, especially for people with a history of relatively mild knee symptoms that haven't improved with exercise, drugs or other treatments. The procedure can be used to smooth out irregular cartilage surfaces, remove chunks of cartilage or bone spurs that have broken off and become loose in the knee joint, or trim away uneven edges of ligaments that fray or tear.

Arthroscopy can be performed under local anaesthesia, and patients generally go home the same day. Full recovery occurs in two to four weeks, sometimes even faster. Pain relief from arthroscopy typically lasts only two to three years – far briefer than that from total joint-replacement surgery. But for those who can't afford the long convalescence that joint replacement requires, arthroscopy might be the solution.

Osteotomy Misalignments of the hip or knee bones can lead to osteoarthritis or make it worse. This may call for osteotomy – a surgical procedure that involves cutting wedges of bone from one or both of the weight-bearing bones of the joint; this has the effect of correcting the misalignment and shifting the body's weight on to the remaining healthy cartilage. Knee osteotomy requires only a day or two in hospital; hip osteotomy requires a somewhat longer stay. Full recovery takes four to six months.

Osteotomy is most effective when the misalignment has caused cartilage to erode in just one area of the joint. The procedure can usually relieve symptoms for an average of seven to 10 years. Osteotomies are especially helpful for very young, active patients with a crooked hip or knee. For them, osteotomy can help to prevent osteoarthritis or postpone the need for joint replacement until they're middle-aged or older.

Synovectomy In this procedure – usually reserved for RA patients and mostly performed on the knee – surgeons remove inflamed synovium, the tissue that forms the inner lining of the joint. The synovium is the target of inflammation, and removing it can prevent it from damaging the joint's cartilage and bone.

Another benefit of removing inflamed synovial tissue is a reduction in joint pain and inflammation. Unfortunately, synovectomy is not a permanent cure, since it is difficult to remove all the synovial tissue – and it can grow back.

Arthrodesis Also known as joint fusion, this procedure is best performed on smaller joints, such as fingers or toes, that have become damaged and unstable – usually because of RA. The joint is rendered permanently immobile through the use of metal screws or a special plaster, reducing pain. The procedure is especially successful on wrist joints, relieving pain while still allowing good use of the hand, and also on ankles.

Forefoot reconstruction This is one of the oldest and most effective surgical procedures for patients who have rheumatoid arthritis – and one of the few operations in which a good result is

Surgery without the glue

Hip replacements can now be performed without cement, especially in people under the age of 60 who have normal bones. The cementless parts of the artificial joint have a very bumpy surface, into which the patient's bones grow – anchoring it in place naturally.

A drawback The bones of some older patients suffering from osteoporosis may not be able to bond well with this kind of artificial joint because their bones are simply not strong enough.

virtually guaranteed. It is performed when most or all of a patient's metatarsophalangeal joints (the ones connecting the toes to the foot) have become severely damaged. The surgeon cuts out the affected joints, leaving soft tissue where the joints were, but providing a surprisingly stable platform on which to walk.

New surgical procedures

Autologous chondrocyte implantation Once cartilage is damaged, the injury is usually permanent. But a new procedure called autologous chondrocyte implantation (ACI) is able to regenerate cartilage in some cases. ACI is available in the UK at the Royal National Orthopaedic Hospital in Stanmore and at the Agnes Hunt and Robert Jones Orthopaedic Hospital in Oswestry.

How it works First, a tiny chunk of cartilage, containing several thousand chondrocytes (cartilage-producing cells), is removed from the patient's healthy cartilage and sent to a laboratory where it is cultured in a petri dish. The cartilage cells are allowed to multiply until about 100 million are present.

The lab then freezes the cells and sends them back to the patient's physician, who reinserts the cartilage by opening the knee joint surgically, patching it, then injecting the new cartilage through the patch into the damaged area.

After the knee is sewn back up, it is stabilized in a brace while the new cartilage takes hold. Since the implanted cartilage is the patient's own and there is no risk that the immune system will reject it and the procedure is proving highly successful.

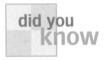

did you know

There is some speculation that the success of ACI may be improved by rapidly transplanting the cultured chondrocytes into the defective cartilage. This can be done by culturing the cells in a location near the operating room, avoiding the delay of having them transported from elsewhere.

Unfortunately, it is also very expensive (about £7,000), and so far it is only considered suitable for a select group of patients who have specific knee injuries or cartilage defects, but may eventually prove useful for treating cartilage loss in oseoarthritis.

Pain-relief strategies: tried and trusted remedies

Amid all the dramatic news about arthritis breakthroughs, people tend to overlook some of the older, simpler but nonetheless helpful treatments available for osteoarthritis and rheumatoid arthritis. Foremost among these old standbys are heat, cold and topical rubs.

Heat or cold?
Knowing when to use what

Many people with arthritis can achieve temporary pain relief by using heat or cold. Heat works better for relaxing muscles and for soothing chronic aches and pain, while cold is the better treatment when arthritic joints are acutely swollen or inflamed.

Some joints like it hot Heat helps to stimulate blood circulation and is a great way to relax stiff muscles or muscle spasms, and soothe aching joints. People generally find more joint-pain relief with moist heat than with dry – probably because moist heat does a better job of warming the tissues underlying the skin. Moist heat in the form of a hot bath is one of the oldest of all treatments for the pain of arthritis.

Ordinary superficial heat – the kind produced by a warm bath or a heating pad – works best for joints closer to the skin surface such as the knuckles and other joints of the hands. For this reason, people with

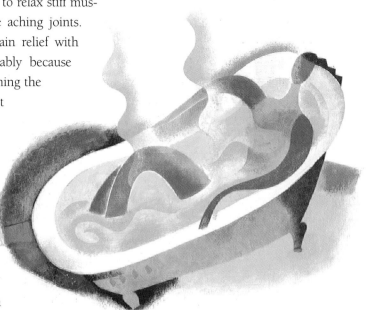

Tips for using heat and cold

◯ You can use heat or cold several times during the day, but don't apply either one to an area for more than 15 or 20 minutes at a time.

◯ Be sure to put a towel or some other barrier between your skin and the source of cold or heat.

◯ Never use heat treatment together with Deep Heat, Ralgex or any other topical pain-relief product as the combination could cause a burn.

◯ Because any form of heat can potentially cause burns, people with diabetes, poor circulation or any other health problem that impairs sensation should be especially careful not to overuse heat.

◯ Check your skin regularly when using heat or cold to prevent frostbite or burns.

◯ When using a heating pad, stick to the low and medium settings and avoid high.

osteoarthritis of the hands may find they obtain quite significant pain relief by immersing their hands in hot water or by using heated mittens.

Getting heat to reach deeper joints, such as the hip or knee, requires use of heat treatments, in which heat is generated by devices that emit shortwave, microwave or ultrasound radiation. (Ultrasound penetrates more deeply than microwave or short-wave radiation.) These treatments are usually available only in a doctor's surgery or in clinics and can be expensive.

The comforts of coolness Cold is better for joints that are acutely painful or inflamed as in rheumatoid arthritis. Applying cold can be useful after exercise, since it can reduce the swelling and muscle ache that may follow a strenuous workout.

How it works Cold has both anti-inflammatory and pain-relieving properties. It can help to numb a painful area, and by reducing the swelling that interferes with healing, can speed up recovery from 'overuse injuries' such as tennis elbow or shin splints. You can quickly make an ice pack by filling a small resealable plastic bag with ice. If ice isn't handy, improvise by wrapping a bag of frozen vegetables or a cold can of soft drink in a towel and applying your 'veggie' or 'cola' pack to a painful joint.

Running hot and cold Some people find that alternating heat and cold treatments provides better relief for arthritis pain than using either of them alone. For example, you can apply a heating pad for 3 or 4 minutes, let your joint rest for a minute, and apply an ice pack for 1 minute. Then repeat the cycle several times – ending the routine with warmth.

Topical pain relievers

Imagine rubbing aspirin or other NSAIDs directly into a painful joint without having to swallow a tablet or capsule. Ideally, you would get the same pain relief that NSAIDs provide – but without the stomach irritation they can cause. Such topical drugs are known as rubefacients. They provide temporary but noticeable pain relief with much less risk of encountering the sometimes serious side effects that oral NSAIDs can cause.

Pain-relieving rubs are marketed under many brand names and with many different ingredients. However, they fall into three main categories: salicylate ointments, capsaicin ointments and counter-irritant ointments that contain one or more substances such as menthol, camphor or eucalyptus.

The salicylate products You may be familiar with topical pain relievers such as Deep Heat and Dubam cream. Like many other nonprescription products, these contain salicylates, a family of drugs that reduces pain and inflammation and that includes acetylsalicylic acid, the active ingredient in aspirin.

How they work Rub-on salicylates are used not only for minor arthritic pain (usually the fingers, knuckles, elbows and knees) but also for strains, sprains, tendinitis and sports injuries. The main ingredient is methyl salicylate and the ointment or cream is usually applied one to three times a day. They may relieve pain in several possible ways:

▶ When rubbed on, salicylates travel a short distance (about three or four millimetres) beneath the skin, perhaps just far enough for some of the ingredient to penetrate directly into a sore joint.

Plug in to a stimulating therapy

Electrical stimulation is the application of small doses of electricity to painful joints and supporting structures. In medical jargon, it is officially known as transcutaneous electrical nerve stimulation, or TENS for short.

How it works Electrodes are coated with a gel and attached to the skin on or near the painful area. The electrodes are attached by wires to the TENS unit, which sends low-level electricity into the skin (using a 9V battery) through the wires and electrodes. Patients may feel a tingling sensation or nothing at all.

Is it effective? Studies in treating arthritis pain have yielded conflicting results. In rheumatoid arthritis patients, studies show that TENS can reduce pain and improve flexibility; in osteoarthritis patients, the results are mixed.

Pain relief from TENS may last only as long as the treatment or for several hours afterward. One advantage is that patients can use TENS therapy at home after they have been instructed in its use. However, people with cardiac pacemakers should never use a TENS unit since the electrical impulses could interfere with the pacemaker's function.

● When salicylates are rubbed into the skin, measurable amounts are absorbed into the bloodstream and may reach the joint that way. In one study, subjects were asked to rub a methyl salicylate product on a large joint four times a day. Researchers found that the equivalent of two aspirin tablets had been absorbed into the bloodstream.

● Adverts for rubs often claim a penetrating heat. Some experts contend that they are effective because the warming sensation distracts users from their joint pain.

Capsaicin products Topical products for arthritis pain in this class contain capsaicin, the chemical responsible for the 'hotness' of red pepper and cayenne. There are many nonprescription creams available; brand-name products include Fiery Jack and Ralgex Stick. Zacin contains 0.025 per cent capsaicin but is available only on prescription.

As well as arthritic pain, capsaicin products are regularly used to relieve other painful conditions, including shingles and post-mastectomy pain.

How they work Most experts believe capsaicin products are more effective than salicylates in relieving minor arthritis pain. One reason for this is that experts have a clearer idea of how capsaicin works. It appears to dull pain by 'robbing' sensory neurons (the nerves that signal pain, touch and other sensations) of substance P – a chemical that is responsible for transmitting the pain felt in various arthritic conditions to the brain. In addition, capsaicin may trigger the release of endorphins, the body's natural pain relievers.

Capsaicin is considered particularly useful against osteoarthritis of the fingers, wrists, hands and knees. But to be effective, these products must be applied frequently; a minimum of four times a day.

People generally notice improvement after applying capsaicin cream for three to seven days. For the first seven to 10 days of use, you may feel significant localized stinging or burning that usually fades after a week or two of regular use.

> **caution**
>
> Apply capsaicin cream with a surgical glove to minimize contact with the skin, and keep it away from the eyes and other sensitive tissues. You should also never use capsaicin products on broken or irritated skin or in combination with a heating pad as this may cause burns.

> ◑ **FACT** Capsaicin takes at least a few days and as much as a month before it really has any effect. This delay in relief may be due to the time it takes to deplete substance P from nerve endings.

There can be an enormous price variation between capsaicin products. As an example, Ralgex Stick costs £4.30 for 50g, while Zacin costs £16.71 for 50g.

In this case the price difference is largely due to the fact that Zacin, being a prescription-only drug, has had a lot of money invested in it in terms of research and development. Zacin should do what it claims to do. But other products containing capsaicin may still be effective.

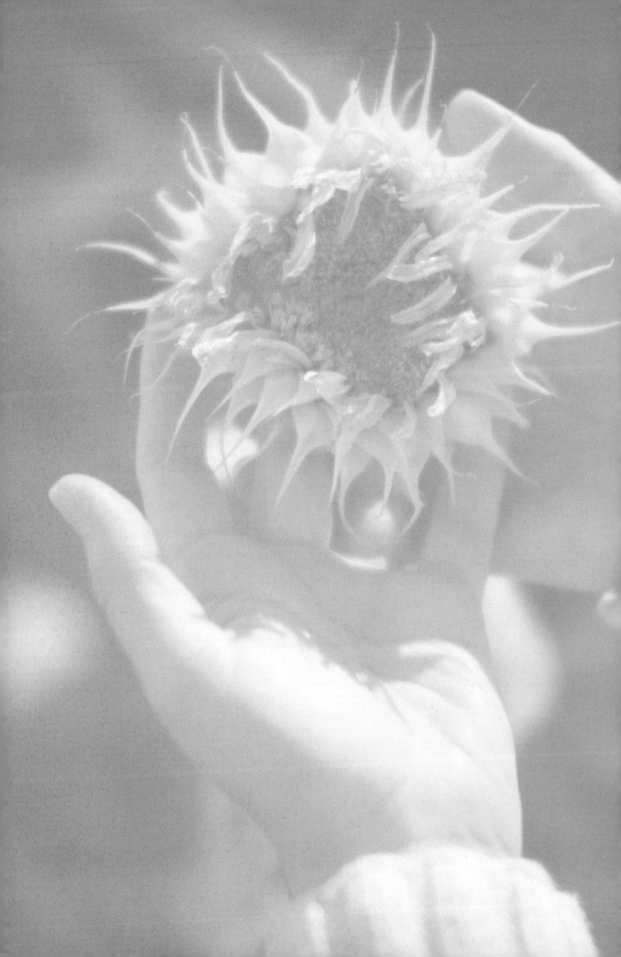

6

Alternative therapies

Opting for alternative

therapies has obvious attractions

for people who want to take charge

of their arthritis. But it is best to

be cautious and do your homework;

alternative medicine can be helpful

but it is not entirely risk free.

Alternative therapies have gone mainstream

At one time, they were exiled to the fringes of medicine, but alternative therapies are now a major part of its fabric. In fact, most sufferers from arthritis will resort to a nonconventional remedy at least once. Consider these facts about alternative therapies and therapists in the United Kingdom.

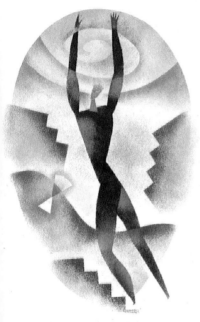

ALTERNATIVE THERAPIES
offer self-empowered patients another avenue to gain control of their disease. Always weigh the evidence of a therapy before trying it.

- The UK has 40,000-50,000 complementary or alternative therapists, who are members of professional groups.

- About 30 per cent of the population has used, or is using, some form of complementary medicine. This rises to 60 per cent among arthritis sufferers.

- HRH The Prince of Wales, in his capacity as President of the Foundation for Integrated Medicine, wrote in 1999: 'A recent BBC poll (of 1,200 people) revealed that one in five Britons now opts to use complementary therapies. Nearly 80 per cent of those asked believed that these therapies were becoming increasingly popular'.

- A recent Department of Health study found that the most common complaints taken to complementary practitioners were problems with persistent pain. This is an area which conventional medicine finds difficult to manage.

Alternatives and arthritis It is rather difficult to compare conventional medicine with complementary therapies. Most medical and other healthcare training institutions in the UK provide little instruction in complementary therapies; similarly, most complementary therapy courses offer little training in conventional medicine. As a result, there are not many examples of complementary therapies and conventional medicine working together. All the more reason for you to make informed decisions.

Proceed with caution

Many arthritis patients have been let down by remedies that promised the moon but succeeded only in depleting their wallets and, in some cases, endangering their health. By following these guidelines, you can help to ensure that alternative treatments won't create more problems than the symptoms you are trying to overcome.

- ◉ Since symptoms of arthritis wax and wane, be careful about crediting an alternative remedy for improvements in your health that might have occurred anyway.

- ◉ Because herbs and other alternative remedies are 'natural' does not mean they are harmless. Many of today's prescription drugs were originally isolated from plants. Herbs can be potent and it is best to consult your doctor before using them as some may have side effects or may interract adversely with a drug you are already taking. Always seek medical advice if side effects occur.

- ◉ Read the label carefully. Food supplement manufacturers must – by law – describe, advertise and present their products accurately. Although the quality of ingredients has not been monitored in the past, new purity criteria for vitamin and mineral ingredients are coming into force.

- ◉ Avoid any alternative therapies that are supported only by testimonials – make sure there has been scientific research.

- ◉ If you're pregnant or breastfeeding, check with your doctor before taking a dietary supplement for arthritis.

- ◉ Beware of alternative therapists who claim 'secret' cures or knowledge – ethical practitioners don't deal in secrets.

Many arthritis patients have eagerly embraced alternative therapies. A recent survey concluded that two-thirds of them have at least experimented with alternative remedies, and many use such treatments regularly. There are certainly a lot to choose from.

◗ **FACT** Use alternative therapies to supplement rather than replace standard treatments such as prescription drugs, weight-loss programmes and exercise.

Hundreds of alternative treatments have been promoted for treating arthritis. Unfortunately, only a handful of these remedies have been studied thoroughly enough to determine whether they are safe and effective.

This chapter offers guidance to those arthritis patients who want to use the most promising alternative treatments wisely and effectively. The focus is mainly on treatments that are currently topical (for example, glucosamine, chondroitin sulphate and SAM), widely used by arthritis patients (acupuncture and chiropractic), especially promising (collagen II supplements for rheumatoid arthritis) or widely recognized as arthritis relief alternatives (copper bracelets).

Hands-on therapies: good for body and mood

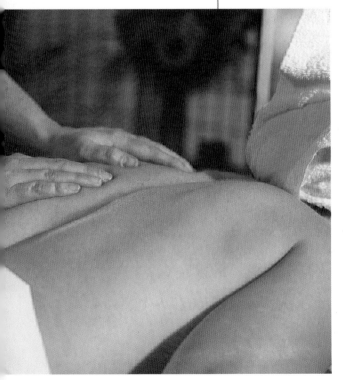

The touch of human hands can help to relieve musculoskeletal pain and emotional distress – a natural consequence of trying to manage a chronic disease like arthritis. With any form of bodywork, success depends on the training, skill and experience of the practitioner. If there is no improvement, try another technique or practitioner.

Massage – touch therapy

The first written references to massage date to about 2000 BC – but in all likelihood, its use probably extends back to prehistory.

One proponent of massage therapy was Hippocrates, who believed that this therapy restored the body's nutritive fluids to their natural free movement.

How it works Massage therapy can help people with arthritis in several ways. It can relax muscles and decrease muscle stiffness and spasm; it decreases pain; it can also increase the range of mobility of the joints. (Interestingly, research has shown that one of the benefits long claimed for massage – increased blood-flow to the muscles – does not actually occur.)

> 'There are few people who would dispute the short-term benefits of massage, for certain types of pain relief where muscle spasm is prominent.'
>
> – Dr. Tom Palferman, consultant rheumatologist, British Society for Rheumatology.

Anyone seeking massage therapy can choose from more than 100 different types, ranging from gentle touching like the Alexander technique to deep-massage techniques such as rolfing and neuromuscular massage.

Massage therapy can be administered by masseurs (most of whom are trained in many of these techniques) as well as physiotherapists, chiropractors and physicians. Or, if you are determined to take charge of your own arthritis, you can do it yourself (see *Do-It-Yourself Massage*, next page).

> ⊙ **FACT** Massage is not usually covered by private medical insurance, unless it is part of a necessary physiotherapy programme.

A massage menu

There is more than one way to decrease pain and relax muscles. Here is a list of some massage or bodywork treatments:

Neuromuscular therapy (NMT) uses precisely focused, calibrated pressure to relax areas of tension or pain that may be contributing to pain in other parts of the body, and ease tense muscles that may be pulling joints out of position. Competent NMT practitioners should have a thorough knowledge of human anatomy and be able to recommend therapeutic exercises.

Rolfing is similar to neuromuscular therapy. Developed more than 50 years ago by Dr. Ida P Rolf, the aim of this therapy is to normalize posture and joint function by relaxing muscles that are tight and contracted. But there is a difference; rolfing focuses on loosening muscles and connective tissues that have adhered to bone structures.

Do-it-yourself massage

Massaging yourself may not be as satisfying as massage done by a professional, but it can make you feel better. Tense muscles can aggravate arthritis pain, and kneading the muscles – especially those around sore joints – can help. Muscles in the neck, arms, fingers, shoulders, thighs and legs are all accessible to self-massagers. Here are some tips for doing your own massage:

- Apply baby powder or baby oil to the area before massaging – it helps to reduce friction and makes it easier to work your muscles.

- Try a variety of different movements, including firm stroking with the palm and fingers, kneading (by 'cupping' muscles between the palm and fingers or squeezing with the thumb and fingers), and making circles with the heel of your hand or your fingertips.

- Don't massage the same spot for more than about 15 or 20 seconds.

- A vibrating massager may be useful for areas that are not easily accessible.

- Don't massage a joint that is severely inflamed or where the skin is irritated, and stop if the massage causes pain.

Shiatsu uses focused finger-pressure to ease pain and stiffness. Like acupuncture and acupressure, it is based on the belief that the fingers can direct therapeutic energy to ailing tissues and organs.

Feldenkrais practitioners teach people how to walk, sit and work in ways that help to restore joint-friendly posture and balance.

Yoga can help to improve your range of movement and strengthen muscles around joints. In one clinical trial, 17 people with osteoarthritis of the hands used yoga to help to relieve pain. Compared with patients who did no yoga, those who practised it ended the experiment with less pain and greater range of movement in the afflicted joints.

Manipulation: pain relief with a twist

Manipulation involves twisting, thrusting or pressing the body. The treatment can help to relieve some types of pain, and it works better than stretching to increase the joint's range of movement.

Several types of healthcare professionals use manipulation in their practice, including osteopaths, physiotherapists and – most notably – chiropractors, who emphasize manipulation of the spine. With its focus on drugless healing and general well-being, chiropractic has benefited from the public's growing interest in alternative medicine.

Doctors and physiotherapists may also use manipulation techniques that are similar to those used by osteopaths and chiropractors. One survey of patients attending a rheumatism clinic in London, found that manipulation was the most helpful of the complementary medical treatments they had tried. But does spinal manipulation – by chiropractors or anyone else – actually help in treating arthritis?

Some two dozen controlled clinical studies have investigated spinal manipulation for a variety of health problems which do not include osteoarthritis. So far, spinal manipulation has been found

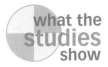
what the studies show

▷ A few years ago, the US magazine, *Consumer Reports* surveyed more than 46,000 readers on their use of alternative therapies. Among readers with arthritis who had received chiropractic care, around 25 per cent reported feeling 'much better' after the treatment, but nearly 40 per cent said chiropractic care had 'helped only a little or not at all'.

Chiropractic do's and don'ts

If you decide to see a chiropractor keep the following points in mind:

● Be wary of claims that spinal manipulation can treat health problems in other parts of the body.

● Manipulation is a forceful procedure that – especially when it involves the neck – carries with it a very small but definite risk of injury, including stroke or paralysis. People with arthritis or ankylosing spondylitis should never undergo manipulation of the neck.

● Be sceptical of the need for long-term treatment. The main benefit of manipulation is rapid relief from low-back pain. If you haven't noticed significant improvement after three weeks of treatment, it's unlikely that manipulation will help you.

effective for treating one condition: common acute low-back pain that has lasted for three weeks or less. In addition, recent research suggests that the therapy may be helpful for neck pain.

How it works Treatment for back or neck pain is the main reason that people see chiropractors. Chiropractors understand that manipulating the spine can have an impact on the entire body. Chiropractic theory is based on the notion that small spinal misalignments, known as subluxations, are the cause of numerous health problems ranging from hypertension to ear infections. Chiropractors contend that spinal manipulations (which they call 'adjustments') can correct those misalignments and thereby clear up health problems or, when done regularly, prevent them from recurring. But despite researchers' efforts to pinpoint them, subluxations remain entirely theoretical.

The bottom line Spinal manipulation is a useful therapy for acute low-back pain and possibly for neck pain, but its effectiveness for relieving back pain due to osteoarthritis remains to be proven.

Acupuncture: treatment with a point

A part of the healthcare system of China, acupuncture has been used for more than 2,500 years. It involves stimulating certain points on or just under the skin by inserting very thin needles and then 'manipulating' them, either manually or with electric current.

How it works Acupuncture is based on the idea that an essential life force, known as *qi*, flows through the body along several channels, or meridians. Disease occurs when one or more of these channels becomes blocked. Inserting needles at appropriate sites – the acupuncture points – along the affected channels restores health by enabling *qi* to flow freely again.

> ◗ **FACT** Similar to acupuncture, acupressure uses fingertip pressure instead of needles to help to disperse lactic acid that builds up in muscles. It is a safe technique that you can learn and use on yourself.

In the 1970s there were very few trained acupuncturists in the UK. Today, 2,400 qualified practitioners are registered with the British Acupuncture Council (BAcC). They see an average of 20 patients a week – roughly 1.8 million treatments a year.

The BAcC does not represent all acupuncturists working in this country. There is no statutory regulation as yet, so there is no pressure on an acupuncturist to register with the BAcC.

Some controversy Despite its popularity, acupuncture remains controversial. Many Western physicians continue to argue that acupuncture has no rational basis, since the meridians it acts upon have never been detected. Acupuncture's effectiveness, they say, can be explained simply by the placebo effect (patients' expectation that a treatment will work) or by distraction (diverting patients' attention from their symptoms by irritating or stimulating another part of the body).

Acupuncture is receiving well-deserved attention as a result of the establishment of the Acupuncture Regulatory Working Group (ARWG) which has been established under the chairmanship of Lord Chan of Oxton. This is a direct response to a commitment made by the health ministers to the House of Lords Science and Technology Committee that the acupuncture profession would be statutorily regulated as soon as practicable. Membership of the ARWG is drawn from the four major voluntary regulatory bodies for acupuncture and, in addition, the Department of Health and the Prince of Wales's Foundation for Integrated Health have observer status. The group aims to examine the options for achieving the successful statutory regulation of the profession as a whole.

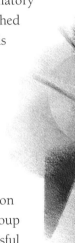

What does it help?

The NHS Direct on-line service lists a number of conditions that might be especially helped by treatment by acupuncture. It says that there is good evidence that acupuncture is an effective treatment for joint pain caused by osteoarthritis, menopausal symptoms, chronic lower back pain and other persistent pain. It states that there is some evidence that acupuncture may help people who suffer from fibromyalgia, tension headaches, neck pain, irritable bowel syndrome, period pain and migraine, but results are less certain.

'One of the advantages of acupuncture is that the incidence of adverse effects is substantially lower than that of many drugs or other accepted medical procedures used for the same conditions.'

– The USA's National Institutes of Health (NIH) Panel on Acupuncture, 1997

The BAcC is the leading body of professional acupuncturists, all of whom have undergone three years' full-time professional training – or the part-time equivalent – and members are subject to a code of ethics and a code of practice. The training is recommended regardless of a person's prior biomedical qualification. The BAcC does not consider it adequate for a provider of acupuncture to have undergone a shorter course in acupuncture, and is working towards statutory regulation of the profession. The BAcC website provides facilities to search for a complete list of practitioners in the UK or in your local area. Visit it at www.acupuncture.org.uk or telephone BAcC on 020 8735 0400.

The bottom line People with osteoarthritis and other forms of arthritis may want to try acupuncture, especially if other treatments haven't helped. You can expect to pay more for the first session (from £40 to £70) because that is when diagnosis takes place and it therefore usually lasts longer. Subsequent appointments can cost from £25 to £60. If you don't notice improvement in your condition after six treatments, then the therapy is probably not going to work for you.

Dietary supplements: therapy you can swallow

Supplements for treating arthritis and other health problems are regulated as foods and are subject to the general provisions of the Trades Description Act 1968, the Food Safety Act 1990 and the Food Labelling Regulations.

The Food Safety Act ensures that foods – and food supplements – are safe to take, are of the quality the consumer is led to expect, and are not misleadingly decribed or labelled. The Food Labelling Regulations make sure that medicinal claims are not made for foods, and that any claims that the supplement contains vitamins or minerals are well founded. These rules also prevent any food supplement from claiming that it can prevent, cure or treat any human disease. If this type of medical claim is made, the substance has to be registered as a medicine, and needs to be licensed by the Medicines Control Agency (MCA). If there are serious problems with a particular dietary supplement, the MCA can take action, in conjunction with the Food Standards Agency.

Choose wisely Like other foods, food supplements are not required to demonstrate their efficacy before being marketed and are not subject to prior approval unless they are novel in some way or genetically modified. It is the responsibility of the manufacturer or importer to ensure that the product complies with UK legislation but food law enforcement officers do have powers to check products for compliance.

To improve the odds that the products you buy will be both effective and safe to use, it may be better to buy supplements from large, reputable manufacturers who distribute their products nationally. In the USA, studies that have analysed dietary supplements suggest that bigger companies generally have a higher level of quality control than smaller firms.

Glucosamine and chondroitin: hope in a bottle

The dietary supplements glucosamine and chondroitin gained almost overnight fame in the USA in 1997, when they were mentioned in *The Arthritis Cure,* a bestseller written by Dr. Jason Theodosakis of the University of Arizona College of Medicine. The book described some 30 clinical studies – mainly from Europe – that found that glucosamine (made from crab shells) and chondroitin (made mainly from cow tracheas) were helpful against osteoarthritis.

Promising research The studies generally showed that glucosamine and chondroitin work significantly better than placebos in relieving pain and improving the mobility of osteoarthritis patients. In addition, the supplements worked at least as well as non-steroidal anti-inflammatory drugs (NSAIDs) such as ibuprofen, and each appeared quite safe, with very few side effects observed.

NSAIDs and other drugs currently used to treat OA can only help to relieve symptoms – and the NSAIDs in particular can cause serious side effects, especially when taken for long periods.

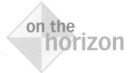

on the horizon

An American-sponsored study is investigating glucosamine and chondroitin sulphate as treatments for OA of the knee. Sponsored by the National Institutes of Health, in the USA, the £4 million double-blind, placebo-controlled study involves more than 1,200 patients and is being carried out at several medical centres around the USA. Patients are randomly assigned to take either glucosamine, chondroitin sulphate, a combination of glucosamine and chondroitin sulphate, a non-steroidal anti-inflammatory drug or a placebo. Results are expected in 2005.

A consumer's guide: what you should know before taking it

● Studies show that it typically takes a month before users of glucosamine and chondroitin notice any benefit, versus one or two weeks for NSAIDs. If you don't notice improvement after about two months, these supplements probably are not for you.

● Glucosamine hydrocholoride is a more concentrated form of the substance and may be more effective than glucosamine sulphate. However, in the UK, the sulphate form is more generally available although glucosamine hydrochloride can be bought from the internet.

● Most of the clinical trials involving glucosamine and chondroitin used daily doses of 1,200mg of chondroitin sulphate and 1,500mg of glucosamine sulphate.

● Diabetics may want to avoid glucosamine or have their blood-sugar levels tested more frequently because animal studies have suggested that glucosamine may worsen insulin resistance.

● People who have a bleeding disorder or are taking a blood thinner (anticoagulant) should be aware that chondroitin sulphate also has an anticoagulant effect.

That explains the increasing public interest in glucosamine and chondroitin sulphate, which seem to be just as effective as certain NSAIDs but much safer.

How they work When glucosamine and chondroitin are swallowed, they are absorbed into the bloodstream and work their biochemical benefits in the joints. It's still not clear just how these two supplements relieve the symptoms of osteoarthritis, but evidence suggests that they may slow the progression of cartilage loss – and may even help to rebuild cartilage that has started to break down. In the joints of the human body, glucosamine and chondroitin are important building blocks of cartilage – particularly of the proteoglycans, the large molecules that give cartilage its resilience. Taking glucosamine as a dietary supplement appears to combat osteoarthritis by stimulating the chondrocytes (cells that manufacture cartilage) to produce more cartilage; chondroitin seems to help to counteract osteoarthritis by interfering with enzymes that degrade cartilage.

Glucosamine sulphate and chondroitin sulphate can be bought individually or as combination supplements. Although, in theory, combinations should be more useful than single-ingredient products, most of the clinical trials have tested glucosamine or chondroitin individually rather than in combination.

So far, all the studies carried out in the US on glucosamine combined with chondroitin have involved one brand, Cosamin DS. Results of two placebo-controlled clinical trials were recently reported – one involving 34 men from the US Navy's amphibious strike unit who had osteoarthritis of the knee or lower back, the other involving 100 patients with OA of the knee. In both studies, patients taking the supplements generally experienced more pain relief than patients in the placebo group.

The bottom line Both glucosamine and chondroitin sulphate show promise in treating osteoarthritis. More studies are needed to prove their effectiveness, but they do seem to relieve the symptoms of OA while posing relatively few risks. Since they don't seem to interact with other OA drugs such as NSAIDs, they may allow you to cut back on the NSAID dose you now take. But be sure to consult your doctor before changing your dosage.

A substance that improves both cartilage and mood?

SAM (known as SAM-e in the USA) is the abbreviated name of s-adenosylmethionine, a chemical found naturally in all cells of the body. It plays a role in many biological reactions – in fact, it appears to regulate more than 30 different mechanisms – and SAM deficiencies have been linked to several neurological disorders, including Parkinson's and Alzheimer's disease.

In the late 1970s, Italian researchers studying SAM's effectiveness as an antidepressant noticed an unexpected side effect: some of their patients said the supplement helped to relieve their arthritis pain. In the United States today, SAM is now one of the most popular dietary supplements, promoted not only for its ability to relieve depression but as a treatment

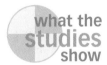
what the studies show

▶ Which is more effective – glucosamine or chondroitin? The jury is still out, and opinions vary. In the US, the *Journal of the American Medical Association* believes chondroitin sulphate is somewhat more effective, but in the UK, the Arthritis Research Campaign favours glucosamine sulphate, saying that there is more evidence in its favour.

for osteoarthritis as well. SAM does appear helpful for both problems, although there is generally more clinical evidence for efficacy against depression than for OA. But the Arthritis Research Campaign points out that, in the UK, there is as yet, no clinical evidence to support the claims made for SAM.

How it works? Research elsewhere has not yet shown how SAM works to relieve the pain of OA. Some evidence from laboratory and animal studies suggests that it may help to rebuild damaged cartilage, but more research is needed to establish this action. Some preliminary studies suggest that SAM may have a disease-modifying effect on osteoarthritis. However, until there is clear clinical evidence, it is wise to be wary.

> ▶ **FACT** Normally, the body manufactures all the **SAM** it needs from the amino acid methionine, which is found in common foods, including meats, soya beans, eggs, seeds and lentils. However, a deficiency of methionine, choline, vitamin B_{12} or folic acid can disrupt the body's ability to produce **SAM.**

As with glucosamine and chondroitin, SAM's efficacy as a treatment for osteoarthritis has been studied mainly in Europe. Some ten clinical trials have indicated that SAM works as well as NSAIDs and better than placebos at relieving the pain of osteoarthritis. (There is no evidence that it can help to combat rheumatoid arthritis.)

In one study in the mid 1980s, 734 patients with OA of the hip, knee, spine or hand were assigned to take a daily dose of either 1,200mg of SAM or 750mg of the NSAID naproxen

High cost – and the dosage?

SAM is not readily available in the UK, but may be ordered from the internet. It is one of the most expensive of all dietary supplements – especially if bought in sufficient quantities to relieve arthritis pain.

In clinical studies demonstrating the effectiveness of SAM against arthritis pain doses of 1,200mg per day have generally been used. As the more usually recommended dosage of around 400mg a day can cost around £30 to £60 a month, taking enough SAM to effectively combat the pain of osteoarthritis could potentially triple the cost to as much as £180 a month, depending on the product.

In fact, no one should take that high a dose without first consulting their doctor, although the 1,200mg a day of SAM appears to have been well tolerated by patients in the clinical trials.

The bottom line SAM may work as well as NSAIDs to relieve the pain of OA while causing fewer side effects. But its high cost means that SAM is beyond the means of some and as yet, it is not generally recommended in the UK.

(Naprosyn). After one month, patients taking SAM reported a degree of pain relief similar to those taking naproxen and they also experienced fewer side effects.

> **◉ FACT** It is often a few weeks before the benefits of taking **SAM** are felt. **US** doctors recommend starting with the minimum effective dose – 400 to 600mg a day.

Findings from this and other clinical trials persuaded the Arthritis Foundation in the United States of SAM's usefulness. In 1999, the foundation issued a statement on SAM noting that its medical experts 'feel that there is sufficient information to support the claim that SAM provides pain relief'.

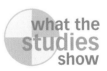

what the studies show

▷ A double-blind study conducted in Germany showed that 36 patients with osteoarthritis who were treated with either SAM or ibuprofen derived the same degree of pain relief.

Collagen supplements: are they in your future?

Type II collagen is cartilage's major protein, providing cartilage with its tensile strength. Research suggests that type II collagen extracted from animals and taken orally can reduce the pain and inflammation of rheumatoid arthritis (perhaps by blunting the misguided immune attack responsible for the disease) while causing minimal side effects.

Promising studies A study published in 1998 involving 60 RA patients found that those taking small doses of chicken collagen for three months experienced significant improvement in swollen and tender joints compared with patients taking a placebo. Similar clinical trials involving small numbers of patients were later carried out, with varying results.

In 2001, scientists at Guy's Hospital in London, carried out a double-blind placebo-controlled clinical trial of type II collagen that found there was a small but significant improvement in disease score in RA in the group given collagen, and there were no side effects. However, they decided that further research was needed into better ways of delivering an accurate dose, in order to induce tolerance and control disease.

You can buy collagen II capsules from the internet, but don't assume that more is better: some clinical studies actually suggest that smaller doses may be more effective than larger ones.

The bottom line Until results of a large-scale study are available, collagen II must be considered a promising but unproven treatment for RA. There is no evidence that it can help people with osteoarthritis. If you do try collagen II supplements, opt for a low daily dose of no more than 60mg.

Cartilage supplements: a no go area

At first glance it makes a lot of sense: since osteoarthritis involves the loss of cartilage from the joints, you can restore the deficit by choosing one of the many cartilage supplements on the market, made from shark, cow, or other animals. But there are no studies to suggest that just any cartilage product will help. True, glucosamine and chondroitin will be found in any cartilage product, but these two ingredients have been found useful only in purified form.

The bottom line It's doubtful that cartilage supplements are of any use in treating arthritis.

Plant and fish oils: modest pain relief

Oils obtained from fatty cold-water fish are rich in omega-3 fatty acids, which have the ability to decrease inflammation. To date, at least 20 clinical studies have shown that high daily doses of fish oil can help to relieve the pain and inflammation of rheumatoid arthritis.

A major evaluation of available studies in 2001 by researchers at Epsom General Hospital and the University of Glasgow concluded that supplementation with fish oils can result 'in a significant reduction in morning stiffness and the number of painful joints in RA patients'. In research, reported in the *Journal of Rheumatology* in February 2000, Spanish researchers concluded that RA patients have a significant deficiency in certain essential fatty acids and suggested that this was why fish and specific plant oils may be beneficial.

In Britain, Professor Bruce Caterson and his team at Cardiff University have recently shown that the omega-3 fatty acids in cod liver oil can also slow – and possibly reverse – the destruction of cartilage that leads to osteoarthritis.

It is best to consult a doctor before taking fish oil supplements if you have high blood cholesterol as therapeutic doses of fish oils are known to raise blood cholesterol levels. Diabetics should also seek medical advice before using fish oils.

Plant power Oils pressed from the seeds of two weedy plants, evening primrose and borage, are rich in the fatty acid gamma linoleic acid (GLA). This fatty acid seems useful against the inflammation of RA, although it hasn't been studied as well as the omega-3s. And GLA is said to raise levels of arachidonic acid (AA) in blood serum – associated with an increased risk of blood clotting, a risk factor for heart disease – although taking fish oils at the same time is reported to offset this effect.

Piascledine – a mixture of oils extracted from avocados and soya beans – can also help to minimize the pain of hip and knee OA, according to two clinical studies from France. In one of the studies, patients with severe OA of the knee or

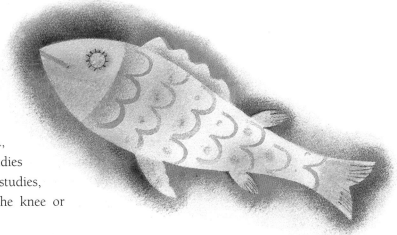

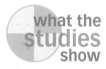

what the studies show

▶ A German study found that taking 1200mg of vitamin E daily decreases pain and morning stiffness and improves grip strength in people with RA as effectively as the drug diclofenac — without stomach upset. However, the British National Formulary (BNF) cautions against taking more than 1000mg a day as it can cause diarrhoea and abdominal pain.

hip who took piascledine experienced less pain and disability after six months than patients taking a placebo. Improvements began after two months without any major side effects. Athough piascledine is not yet sold directly in the UK, it can be bought in France and is now also available in the USA.

How it works Although it is unclear how piascledine works, experts suggest that the oils may prompt chondrocytes (cartilage-making cells) to produce chemicals that help to repair damaged cartilage.

The bottom line RA patients may gain some pain relief by taking fish oils, though there is less evidence for evening primrose oil or borage seed oil (and borage seed oil should only be used under medical supervision – see Caution above, left). In most cases, the supplements may have to be taken for at least three months before they have any noticeable effect. Piascledine may also be helpful in treating osteoarthritis.

The antioxidant advantage: vitamins C, E and beta carotene

Growing evidence indicates that chemicals called free radicals may play a role in causing diseases associated with ageing, including cataracts, heart disease, some types of cancer and osteoarthritis. On the plus side, chemicals called antioxidants – particularly the vitamins C, E and beta carotene that are found in many fruits and vegetables – can neutralize free radicals and prevent them from causing damage.

> ▶ **FACT** Aspirin and other non-steroidal anti-inflammatory agents (NSAIDs) can cause stomach irritation and ulcers; among these, ibuprofen is considered the least likely to produce such adverse side effects.

Damage control Free radicals form constantly within cells – in the joints and elsewhere – during normal metabolism as cells burn up oxygen to create energy. Studies have shown that these chemicals can damage cartilage and may contribute to the damage that occurs in arthritic joints.

So could eating a diet that is rich in antioxidant vitamins – or taking them in the form of dietary supplements – help you to ward off OA or perhaps at least ease its symptoms? Both long-running and recent studies suggest that the answer is yes.

The famous Framingham Heart Study, in which researchers have followed the residents of Framingham, Massachusetts, for nearly 50 years, has shed light on other health problems besides heart disease. In one study, the Framingham researchers looked for evidence of osteoarthritis of the knee in 640 people who were evaluated during two reviews spaced about ten years apart. The subjects also filled in a questionnaire asking about their dietary intake.

The study found that people who took in more than 180mg of vitamin C a day were only a third as likely as people consuming half that amount to have their OA worsen over ten years – a benefit due mainly to reduced cartilage loss. In addition, people with OA who consumed vitamin C in moderate or high amounts were much less likely to develop knee pain.

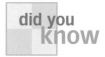

did you know

▶ Bioflavonoids may help to strengthen cartilage and possibly lessen its chances of becoming inflamed. Bioflavonoids are found in virtually all plant foods: fruits, vegetables, pulses, grains and nuts.

Alternative therapies: how to tell your doctor

Don't keep it a secret – tell your doctor about the alternative treatments you use. Herbs and other supplements can cause side effects and dangerous drug interactions, possibly entailing costly tests or treatments, if your doctor doesn't know you've been using them.

In the USA Surveys show that 40 to 60 per cent of American people who use alternative therapies do not disclose that fact to their doctors, presumably for fear of ridicule or criticism. But in Britain, you probably needn't worry, since doctors today are much more accepting of alternative therapies than they were just a few years ago.

A survey in the US magazine *Consumer Reports* found that when people felt comfortable enough to inform their doctors about their alternative choices, a majority of the doctors (55 per cent) expressed approval. Some 40 per cent took a neutral stance, and only 5 per cent disapproved.

caution

People on prescription blood-thinning drugs (anticoagulants) or aspirin should consult their doctor before using vitamin E (which also thins the blood).

A study conducted by researchers at the Arthritis Research Campaign's epidemiology unit at the University of Manchester, in conjunction with the Ministry of Health at the University of Cambridge, confirmed that a low intake of fruit and vegetables – particularly those containing vitamin C – appears to increase the risk of developing inflammatory arthritis.

Some 25,000 people were given health and dietary assessments, between 1993 and 1997. They were followed-up, over an eight-year period, to see which of them developed inflammatory polyarthritis. Over the eight years, 73 cases were identified; it was clear from the research findings that lower intakes of fruit, vegetables, fructose and dietary vitamin C were associated with a greater risk of inflammatory polyarthritis.

Findings for vitamin E and beta carotene in the Framingham tests were also positive, but not quite as impressive as for vitamin C. People consuming the highest amounts of beta carotene had half the risk of seeing their OA worsen compared with people consuming the least amount. And for vitamin E, the benefits were more modest and limited to men: those who consumed the most vitamin E were significantly less likely to have their OA worsen compared with men in the lowest category.

The bottom line It is premature to recommend antioxidant supplements for preventing or treating arthritis – the evidence for benefit comes from too few studies. But if you are concerned that you don't eat the recommended five to nine daily servings of fruit and vegetables, supplementing your diet with vitamin C (the antioxidant that seems most helpful against arthritis) may be a good idea.

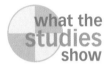

what the studies show

▶ Antioxidants may also help against rheumatoid arthritis. Two small studies have found that people with a low intake of vitamins C, E and beta carotene were more likely to develop RA than people with higher intakes.

Vitamin D: to fortify your bones and cartilage

Vitamin D is essential for healthy bones, since it helps the body to absorb calcium, the key ingredient in bone. But since the bones in a joint are joined to their cartilage, vitamin D could influence osteoarthritis as well.

How it works Researchers believe that a bone's 'integrity' – that is, its ability to withstand weight-bearing activities and other stresses – may affect whether OA worsens or not. So for people with osteoarthritis who also have 'soft' bones – perhaps because

Get your vitamins from foods first

In general, it is best to get as much of the vitamins and minerals you need from your diet, not from a supplement. Foods contain phytochemicals and other potentially beneficial compounds not found in pills that may help in your battle plan against arthritis.

However, if your diet is poor, it may be advisable to add a daily multivitamin/multimineral supplement to your intake to supply missing nutrients. For those on a low-fat diet, it can be difficult to obtain the amount of vitamin E required to benefit from its disease-fighting potential as the vitamin is mainly found in high-fat foods. In this case you may want to consider taking a supplement in capsule or tablet form.

of inadequate vitamin D intake – OA may be a more serious problem. Vitamin D also affects cartilage directly, by stimulating the cells that produce cartilage to make more of it.

Bearing all of this in mind, the Framingham researchers (see page 189) decided to investigate whether dietary vitamin D might influence osteoarthritis. They carried out their study using the same basic methods that they had previously employed in their antioxidant study.

> **◑ FACT** In the West, most dietary vitamin D comes from fortified foods such as margarine – which in Britain is fortified with vitamin D by law – and also from breakfast cereals. In the USA, milk is fortified with vitamin D.

In addition to vitamin D from food, people synthesize their own vitamin D when their skin is exposed to the sun's (and artificial) ultraviolet rays – which is why it is also called the sunshine vitamin. So the researchers assessed not only the vitamin D in people's diets but also – to get a more complete idea of the vitamin's presence – measured the level of D in their blood.

When D becomes toxic

Since vitamin D is a fat-soluble vitamin, it is not excreted readily and can easily build up to toxic levels in your tissues. Too much vitamin D can cause calcium deposits in the body, resulting in serious damage to the kidneys and cardiovascular system.

Play it safe by avoiding vitamin D supplements. There is only a small margin between safe and toxic levels and most of us get all the vitamin D we need from just 10-15 minutes of midday sunlight two or three times a week.

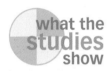
what the studies show

▶ Green tea contains compounds called polyphenols, which may help to relieve RA inflammation. In one study, green tea extract was found to cut the rate of arthritis in animals. Green tea is available in capsules, or can be drunk in the traditional way. Don't add milk to your tea, however – it may block the effects of the beneficial polyphenols.

Persuasive proof Vitamin D was found to have an important influence on OA. People who consumed little vitamin D and had low levels in their serum were three times more likely to experience a worsening of their knee OA than those who had high intakes and high serum levels. In addition, low serum levels of the vitamin were associated with loss of cartilage in the knee.

The bottom line The US evidence suggests that to keep bones and cartilage healthy you should consume at least the Recommended Dietary Amount of vitamin D each day (5mcg), the daily requirement under European Union regulations (their is no UK recommendation); the recommended intake in the USA for people over 50 is 10mcg. You can further boost your levels of vitamin D by getting more sun exposure or by taking a multivitamin containing vitamin D.

Herbal solutions: do your homework

Herbal products have been used for thousands of years to treat virtually every human ailment, including arthritis. But despite the dozens of herbs purported to treat arthritis, patients in the US have largely steered clear of them – at least when it comes to treating their condition.

For example, in its recent survey of alternative-therapy use, the US magazine *Consumer Reports* found that only a small percentage of the arthritis patients who used alternative therapies chose herbal remedies – and the herbs they used such as echinacea, garlic and ginkgo biloba were – surprisingly – not species that are generally used for treating the condition.

> **◐ FACT** Boswellia is a gum derived from a tree native to India. In animal studies, it has been shown to inhibit inflammation and prevent the loss of glycosaminoglycans, which are important components of cartilage.

The bottom line If you are interested in trying herbal remedies for arthritis, be aware that evidence for their effectiveness is almost entirely anecdotal. Herbs that may show some benefit against arthritis and seem reasonably safe include angelica, boswellia, devil's claw, ginger and meadowsweet.

Even if an enthusiastic friend tells you about his or her miraculous experience with one herb or another, resist the seduction; do your homework online or in a library, or check with your doctor first, or consult a qualified medical herbalist, who may be able to offer both advice and treatment. Natural is not synonymous with non-toxic, especially if you are also taking prescription drugs – which can interact dangerously with herbs.

Other treatments: what's hype, what's not

Ever since Neanderthal man woke up with stiff, aching joints, we have been looking for an antidote – standard remedies, alternative approaches, home remedies, anything. Some are reasonable and safe; others don't have a scientific leg to stand on.

Antibiotics: for RA patients only

For types of arthritis that are caused by bacterial infections, antibiotics are a useful treatment. Antibiotics also show promise in easing the inflammation of rheumatoid arthritis – but not for the reasons you might think.

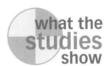

what the studies show

◐ In one study, people with RA showed decreases in pain, stiffness, joint tenderness and swelling, and inflammation, and improvement in grip strength after four months of taking a combination of four plant extracts: boswellia, ginger, curcumin (the active component in turmeric), and *withania somnifera* (also known as ashwagandha).

MSM: the sulphur connection

The dietary supplement MSM (methyl sulfonyl methane) has been promoted for treating arthritis and many other health problems. This sulphur compound is found in a number of foods including milk, fish, grains and fresh fruits and vegetables. Sulphur is an important element in chemicals that make up cartilage – and MSM is destroyed when food is processed – leading proponents to claim (without any scientific support, of course) that MSM is the answer to arthritis problems.

An unproved remedy MSM is sold as a dietary supplement in powder, pill and lotion form. According to Arthritis Care there is no scientific evidence to back the claim that MSM is a cure for arthritis.

Some animal studies are promising, but there have been no human trials, and there is no research to show that it is safe, despite claims that it is non-toxic.

Researchers have long suspected that viruses or other microbes play a role in triggering RA. Yet decades of intensive searching have turned up little evidence to support the notion. As a result, the beneficial effects of minocycline – the antibiotic that seems most useful against RA – apparently have nothing to do with killing bacteria or any other organisms.

How they work When antibiotics are given, many of them can affect human cells – in ways that have nothing to do with their action against microbes. Research on minocycline (which is a member of the tetracycline family of antibiotics) suggests that it muffles the immune response that causes RA, while at the same time suppressing the cells responsible for the destructive enzymes that inflame the joints of RA patients.

The bottom line Three well-regarded clinical trials suggest that minocycline may offer a genuine benefit in treating RA, especially in the early stages of the disease. If you have RA and aren't satisfied with your current therapies, you may want to talk to your doctor about trying minocycline.

Copper bracelets: jewellery, not therapy

Copper's use as a therapeutic agent was noted in an Egyptian papyrus prepared in 1550 BC – and wearing copper bracelets in the hope of combating arthritis pain may date back almost that far. However, there is no good evidence that copper eases the inflammation or pain of arthritis. Actually, copper levels in the blood of RA patients are usually *higher* than normal, casting further doubt on copper's usefulness.

The bottom line By all means wear a copper bracelet if you like its appearance, but don't expect it to ease your arthritis. However, the placebo-effect of believing that it is helping you can do no harm, and may be positively beneficial.

DMSO: risky business

A cleaning fluid similar to turpentine, DMSO (dimethyl sulphoxide) is used mainly as an industrial solvent but has been touted as a treatment for numerous health problems, including arthritis, cancer, mental illness, stroke, multiple sclerosis and varicose veins. The Medicines Control Agency has approved DMSO for treating interstitial cystitis (an uncommon bladder disease), but not for any other medical purposes.

Side effects The chemical has been shown to cause damage to the lens of the eye in animal studies and can be potentially toxic to the liver in humans. The most common side effects are rashes, headache, nausea and diarrhoea.

The bottom line DMSO has not been well studied as an arthritis treatment – and the available evidence provides little assurance that the solvent is either effective or safe.

Magnet therapy: attracting attention

Unless you've been totally out of touch for the past couple of years, you've probably been hearing about 'the healing power of magnets'. They've recently been promoted for their ability to ease the pain of arthritis and carpal tunnel syndrome, heal injuries, improve circulation and provide relief from asthma and other medical problems. But don't throw away your heating pad or ibuprofen. Magnets may be attracting a lot of buyers, but their effectiveness has not been proved beyond doubt.

Magnetic appeal Medical magnets can be bought in sporting goods shops and pro shops at golf courses, through catalogues and from the internet. You can purchase them individually, as thin

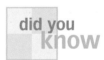

did you **know**

▶ Magnet therapy dates back to the ancient Greeks. Hippocrates reportedly used the magnetic rock lodestone to treat sterility.

strips containing numerous magnets, and in many other forms, including magnetic headbands (for headaches), mattress pads (for arthritic joints and backache), and shoe insoles (for sore feet).

How they work One theory holds that magnets improve blood flow, delivering extra oxygen and nutrients to the area while reducing toxins. The best evidence that magnets offer medical benefits arose from a small study on pain relief carried out at Baylor College of Medicine in Houston, Texas, USA, and published in 1997. It involved 50 people suffering from the pain of postpolio syndrome; 29 of them had magnets placed over their painful areas for 45 minutes, while the other 21 received comparable treatment from sham magnets.

The findings: 76 per cent of the people treated with the real magnets reported a decrease in pain, while only 19 per cent of those treated with sham magnets noticed any improvement. That's a significant difference – but each patient was treated only once, and the study failed to note how long the pain relief lasted.

> ◖ **FACT** There are clear differences in the different brands of magnets on the market. If you try one particular brand and it fails to relieve your pain, try at least two others.

The bottom line So far, no published studies have shown that magnets can ease the pain of osteoarthritis or any other type of arthritis. On the other hand, magnets are relatively inexpensive and – unless you have an electronic pacemaker – apparently safe to use. So if you're drawn to trying magnets for arthritis pain, there's no harm in giving them a try.

Mind over matter: short-circuiting stress

You were going to go visit a friend today, but thanks to the flare-up of knee pain when you woke up, you'll have to let your friend down. What you may not know is that the anger, anxiety and frustration you feel may well be exacerbating your pain, making it even worse.

Just relax: techniques to reduce the tension

The stress response When pain is a chronic problem, stress can become chronic, too – and it can make bad arthritis even worse. How? Stress can lower your pain threshold and can cause muscles around the joints to tighten, literally squeezing them and limiting their range of movement.

However, you don't have to put up with the painful fall-out of stress. You can, as you have with everything else affecting your condition, take charge. There are proven self-help techniques that can help to defuse tense emotions. In fact, clinical studies have shown that arthritis patients who regularly use such techniques can reduce their pain and improve their mobility. Next time your pain gets the better of your emotions, try one of these relaxing strategies:

Biofeedback This technique vividly illustrates mind over matter, training the mind so that it can learn to control physiological functions such as heart rate and blood pressure. A machine using electrodes attached to your skin records subtle physical processes, such as your pulse rate, heart rate or even the muscular tension you are experiencing. These processes are measured on the biofeedback machine as electrical signals or sounds. With practice, you can learn how to control these internal functions – by changing your thought patterns, for example, or visualizing a pleasant scene, or rationalising your way out of the stressful situation, until you return to normal.

Eventually, as you learn what mental technique produces the desired change, you'll be able to produce those physical changes on your own – without the help of the equipment.

> **◐ FACT** Stress reduction may be especially important for people with rheumatoid arthritis, since studies suggest that stress may worsen symptoms of the disease by disrupting immune function.

Studies show that biofeedback can relieve stress and pain associated with fibromyalgia, rheumatoid arthritis and chronic pain associated with osteoarthritis. Learning to relieve your symptoms this way may take just a few biofeedback sessions or could take twenty or more.

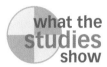

what the studies show

▶ In a study published in 1996, researchers looked at 19 studies comparing NSAID treatment alone for arthritis with treatment that included NSAIDs and mind-body techniques. Compared with NSAID treatment alone, mind-body treatments provided an additional 20 per cent improvement in symptoms for OA patients and an extra 20 to 40 per cent boost for RA patients. Mind-body therapies were especially helpful in improving the functional ability of RA patients and decreasing their number of tender joints.

Visualization This technique channels the power of the imagination to create changes in the body – namely, relieving stress and easing the pain and other symptoms of arthritis. As you recognize yourself getting tense, conjure up a peaceful setting – lying on a tropical beach, for example, or looking out over a sea of sunflowers on a summer's day.

Alternatively, you can visualize yourself doing some desired activity, such as working in the garden, and doing it effortlessly and without pain. Or you can tackle your pain head-on, imagining that the pain is red and hot. Gradually, visualize the colour changing to a cool blue as it fades.

To enhance the results of visualization, choose a quiet, dimly lit room and a time when you can stay there undisturbed.

Guided imagery This is essentially 'visualization' plus – namely, through the aid of a mental health professional or other practitioner who guides you through the mental exercises. The therapist will first put you through exercises to help you to relax and then encourage the sort of visualizations that may help to produce relief for your symptoms.

Meditation This form of relaxation dates back thousands of years to the earliest religions and includes many different techniques. The basic purpose of all meditation techniques is to influence your consciousness by redirecting your attention in some way – focusing on your breathing, for example, or a single word, thought or object, in order to rid your mind of all other thoughts and feelings.

Meditation helps to diminish arthritis symptoms by reducing the stress that exacerbates them. The term 'relaxation response', in fact, grew out of the meditation research of Harvard physician Herbert Benson, who proved that a simple meditation technique (just sitting in a quiet place and focusing on any phrase or sound) can bring about physiological changes, such as lowered heart rate and blood pressure, in almost anyone.

Not surprisingly, the more that you can practise meditation, the better you will get at it – and the more benefits you will achieve. Try meditating at least three or four times a week. Choose a quiet time, when you are unlikely to be disturbed, and make sure you are comfortable and safe, before you start. Don't worry if you fall asleep while meditating.

Beyond relaxation: help for the depressed

Not everyone can be rescued by mind-body therapies. For some people, arthritis can simply be too much to cope with. The stress from their pain and disability creates a level of anxiety, depression or other emotional problems that can only be helped by a mental-health professional. It's understandable that a chronic disease like arthritis should overwhelm you emotionally. Managing it can start to dominate your life – taking medication, keeping doctors' appointments, going online to find out about the latest research or trying new treatments that are not helping your pain.

> ⓒ **FACT** Support groups, either face-to-face or online, are an effective way to deal with the emotional problems caused by arthritis. According to Dr. Ronald C Kessler at Harvard, self-help groups have become one of the most important ways to deal with emotional problems.

Making the call If you feel overwhelmed by your arthritis – and friends and family can't help – there are other options. Your GP can refer you to a professional counsellor who might be able to lift you out of your gloom.

As anyone can call himself a counsellor, it is safest to go through the British Association for Counsellors and Psycho-therapists. This is a registered charity with 20,000 members, all of whom must adhere to the organization's strict regulations. The BACP encourages members to become accredited, which takes three to five years. Their members' list shows whether members are accredited, the form of therapy in which they specialize, as well as their location. One of these approved therapies is cognitive behavioural therapy.

How it works The aim of cognitive behavioural therapy is to get patients to focus on their negative thoughts, and to recognize the link between their negative way of thinking and the stress or depression they're feeling. Once patients realize that their negative attitude is not only distorted but contributes to their emotional turmoil, they may take a more positive approach that helps to lift depression and stress. As with any therapy, a rapport between patient and therapist is essential.

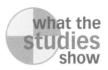

what the studies show

ⓒ A 1998 survey of arthritis patients found that 29 per cent were extremely depressed but that few of them received any intervention for their depression. And studies have found that rates of depression among patients with rheumatoid arthritis are seven times higher than the rate for the general population.

ⓒ A study published in 1999 in the *Journal of the American Medical Association* found that people with mild to moderately severe rheumatoid arthritis could significantly ease their symptoms by writing about their stressful experiences.

7

Eating to beat arthritis

Perhaps the best medicine for

your arthritis isn't something you

get from a chemist or healthfood

shop, but something from the

supermarket shelves. Eating the

right foods has helped many patients

to improve their condition.

Weighty problems

**Being overweight increases your risk of developing
a host of serious conditions such as heart disease,
some cancers, diabetes and, of course, osteoarthritis.
What's more, if you have already been diagnosed
with arthritis and are also overweight, you will suffer
more than slimmer people with the disorder; the
extra pounds can cause further damage to your
joints and worsen pain and stiffness.**

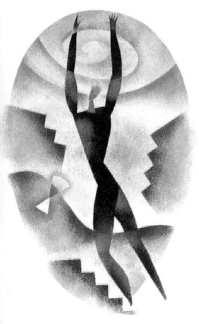

TAKING CHARGE of your
diet enables you to take
charge of your disease
three times a day.
This is especially true
for osteoarthritis
sufferers who are
overweight.

Not surprisingly, losing weight can protect your joints and will
significantly ease your symptoms. But there's much more to
weight control than just calories. Recent studies show that
eating foods rich in certain vitamins and other nutrients can
slow down the progression of osteoarthritis and ward off its
symptoms. Some of these nutrients seem to help to protect the
joints from damage – something that not even drugs can do.

Overweight and OA

Piling on extra pounds is now recognized as a major cause of
osteoarthritis. And judging by recent surveys showing that more
than half of all Britons are overweight – the UK currently has the
eighth-highest obesity rate in the world – it may be the most
important cause of all. In particular, being overweight can cause
OA of the weight-bearing joints – the knees and, to a lesser extent,
the hips. But it is also associated with a greater risk of OA in other
joints as well, including the back, ankles, big toes and hands.

The pressure of pounds When you think about it,
obesity's role in causing OA – or in aggravating symptoms in
people who already have the disease – makes a great deal of
sense. The protective cartilage that covers the ends of the bones
in a joint is just a few millimetres thick. Years of carrying around
extra weight puts extra pressure on the knees and other weight-
bearing joints, grinding down cartilage to the point that bone
rubs against bone and giving rise to the pain and stiffness of OA.
In people who already have OA, being overweight can speed up
cartilage loss and cause the disease to worsen.

Studies have documented the overweight-arthritis link. They have followed groups of people over several years, keeping close checks on their weight and whether they developed OA. One study involved more than 1,000 women aged 45 to 64 who lived in London; 58 of the 67 women with OA in one knee returned for a follow-up X-ray two years later. Of the 32 clearly overweight women, 15 – or nearly half – had by then developed OA in their other knee as well; but only one of the ten normalweight women had gone on to develop OA in the other knee.

The advantages of weight-loss

The good news is that overweight people who lose weight can prevent OA of the knee from occurring. This was first demonstrated in a study published in 1992 – the first ever to show that OA was potentially preventable. And the weight loss didn't need to be dramatic: the study found that by losing just 11lb over a ten-year period, overweight people could reduce their risk of developing OA of the knee by 50 per cent.

The vicious circle When it comes to OA, being overweight is notorious for pushing patients down that long and slippery slope paved with increasingly more severe symptoms. Once people develop arthritis, there are often reasons – many of them totally understandable – why patients continue to put on weight or cannot take it off.

Arthritis sufferers frequently become depressed, which can lead to overeating that adds even more pounds. In addition, someone with stiff, sore joints tends to prefer sitting in front of TV to getting up and going for a brisk walk. That means more weight gain and even worse pain and disability.

Unfortunately, the health impact of gaining too much weight goes beyond arthritis. Being overweight can increase your risk of developing many other health problems as well – high blood pressure, Type 2 diabetes (that is, adult onset diabetes), heart disease and several types of cancer, including prostate cancer and colorectal cancer.

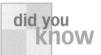

did you
know

▶ The Arthritis Research Campaign is funding a major clinical trial in Nottingham to establish that a combination of weight loss and exercise could help to reduce knee pain in overweight people. If such an exercise and weight-loss programme were implemented nationwide, the savings to the NHS on drugs and knee replacement surgery would be considerable.

did you know

▶ The Arthritis Research Campaign says that a quarter of all cases of osteoarthritis of the knee might be prevented, if only obesity could be eliminated.

Are you overweight?

For most of us, deciding whether we're overweight is painfully easy: a glance in the mirror will usually suffice, and then there are the trousers that are too tight or the collars that no longer button up. Half of our total body fat is wedged between the muscles and the skin, so we can usually sense when there is too much of it. But more scientific methods are also available, including the height-weight chart below.

The chart is intended for use by both men and women and has some wide ranges for each category. Note that people who are the same height can differ by more than 25lb and still fit into the 'healthy weight' range – mainly because two people of the same height can have widely differing amounts of 'heavy' muscle and bone. (Men, with their greater muscle and bone mass, usually weigh more than women of the same height.) The chart is shown in pounds. If you know your weight only in stones, multiply the stones by 14 and add the extra pounds.

Do you weigh too much? (men and women)

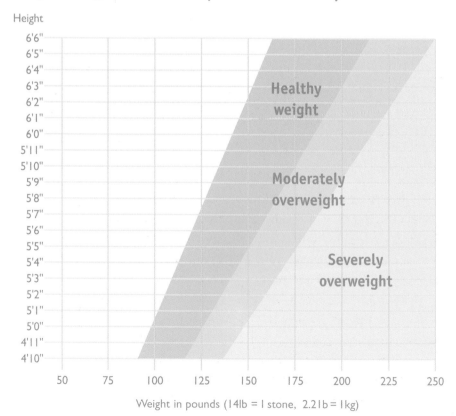

Weight in pounds (14lb = 1 stone, 2.2lb = 1kg)

Weight-loss principles

Many diets fail because they involve dramatic changes that only the most resolute can stick to. The better and more lasting approach is reshaping your eating habits a little at a time. Here are some useful tips:

- Make changes for your own sake, not to please others. You must want to lose weight, keep fit and reduce your osteoarthritis symptoms. You can't do it just because your spouse or your best friend has nagged you into it.

- Record everything you eat to pinpoint your weaknesses. Do it for a week, including the weekend as well.

- Focus on making wise food choices rather than resisting temptation. Very few win the willpower game.

- Don't avoid delicious foods. Instead, satisfy your urges with appealing alternatives such as oven-baked potato chips instead of the deep-fried variety.

- Don't let yourself get too hungry. Skipping one meal leads to overeating at the next. Missing out on breakfast can leave you hungry all day.

- Get at least some exercise everyday. Keeping your body moving raises your metabolic rate so that you burn calories faster than before, even when resting.

Don't assume that you have no problems just because you are within the upper limit of 'healthy'. Even small weight gains within the range of healthy weights may increase your risk of health problems. But if you're muscular, have a large frame and are in good health, then your weight is probably satisfactory.

The height that we achieve as an adult is genetically determined (unless one has suffered severe malnutrition as a child). Our weight, however, is continually influenced by factors such as diet and lifestyle. There is a small genetic influence, but it is extremely small when compared with the choices we make about the food we eat and the amount of exercise we take.

Eat well to live well

Healthy eating involves much more than just adding up long lists of the calories you eat in a day. The idea is not only to lose weight if you need to, but also to eat the right kinds of foods: those that are low in fat and high in beneficial nutrients such as fibre and vitamins.

Ideally, this approach to eating is not only effective but also practical – a new way of eating that you can stick to day after day without feeling either deprived or bored.

Faddy diets come and go, and there is always one which is being touted by super-thin celebrities. However, there is a simple, straightforward way to control and check what you are eating. It involves recognizing the groups into which certain foods fall, and eating the right amount of each group.

In the pyramid-shaped illustration here, you will see the largest group, at the bottom, consists of breads, cereals and other complex carbohydrates. Above them come fruits and vegetables, then meats and fish, milk and other dairy products. The smallest group is made up of sugary, fatty foods. The number of portions of each group that you should eat daily is indicated by its size and position in the pyramid. Later in this chapter, we will talk about the actual size of the portions and how many of each you should eat on a daily or weekly basis. The key to successful weight-loss is, however, simple: balance, variety and moderation.

Losing it for good Sticking to these principles can help people with osteoarthritis to lose weight if necessary and then maintain the healthy weight they have achieved. Equally important, it can help you to ward off or reduce your risk of developing cancer, heart disease, diabetes, hypertension and other health problems associated with being overweight.

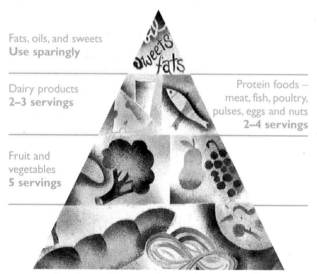

Fats, oils, and sweets
Use sparingly

Dairy products
2–3 servings

Protein foods – meat, fish, poultry, pulses, eggs and nuts
2–4 servings

Fruit and vegetables
5 servings

Bread, cereals, rice, and pasta **6–14 servings**

A guide – not a diet

Although figures vary slightly, researchers have discovered that in the UK, 1 in 5 men and 1 in 3 women (aged between 19 and 64) are currently trying to lose weight. In January 2003 around 12.8 million people in the UK started a diet.

Extensive research and surveys of dieters themselves all show that any commercial diet programme can produce significant weight loss – and even produce it rapidly. But the ultimate goal – especially for OA sufferers – is to keep that weight off, and the vast majority of dieters are not able to do that. Almost inevitably, they regain all the weight they lose on crash diets.

Focus on food The secret of weight-loss success is that you don't follow a diet but, instead use a healthy guide to eating. There is not so much need to focus on calories, but rather think about the food groups that are best for long-term good health: starches, fruits and vegetables. These foods are high in health-promoting vitamins, minerals and other nutrients and low in saturated fat, cholesterol and calories.

> ⊙ **FACT** It is best to get your nutrients
> from whole food rather than supplements.
> Fresh foods contain a host of other beneficial
> substances, such as phytochemicals, that can
> be crucial to reducing arthritis symptoms.

Not surprisingly, following these recommendations will almost inevitably mean reducing your calorie intake and losing weight in the process – and, even better, having an excellent chance of maintaining that weight loss.

Getting it into proportion

If you include the number of portions of different foods that we recommend in your daily intake, you should have little appetite left for crisps and chocolate bars. However, there is enough variety in each food group to keep your diet interesting and varied. The key is to make the right choices within each food group.

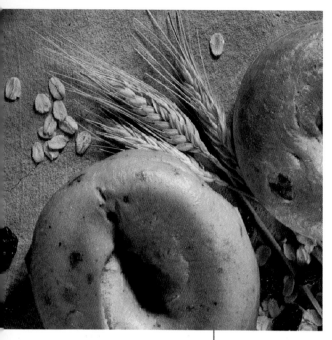

Start with starches

The largest food group consists of starchy carbohydrates – bread, cereal, rice and pasta. Carbohydrates are the foundation of a healthy diet, and should make up at least half the calories in your daily intake.

Contrary to what you may think or have heard, these starches are not fattening – as long as you leave off the butter and other high-fat toppings such as full-fat cheese or sour cream, or sugary jams and spreads. Also, pasta and other starches have the virtue of leaving you feeling satisfied.

Portion sizes You should try to eat 6 to 14 portions a day, most of them from whole-grain varieties. A single portion can be either 1 slice of bread, 3 tablespoons of cereal, a bread roll, bap or bun, 1 small pitta bread, naan bread or chapatti, 3 crackers or crispbreads, a medium-sized potato or half a cup of cooked rice or pasta.

> **◐ FACT** Eat mostly whole grains that are high in fibre. Because most fibre leaves the body undigested, your body doesn't absorb the calories it contains.

Fruit and vegetables

The next largest group of foods in the ideal diet is composed of fruits and vegetables. Both are nature's attempt at diet food – low in fat and calories and rich in flavour, fibre, phytochemicals and antioxidant vitamins that are especially important for anyone suffering with osteoarthritis.

It's not as hard as you might think to make fruits and vegetables a larger part of your diet – and to improve your joints and your overall health in the process. By following these suggestions, you can boost your intake of fruits and vegetables immediately:

◐ Begin your day with 4-6fl oz (125-175ml) of pure fruit juice (a small glass), such as freshly squeezed orange or grapefruit juice.

what the studies show

◐ Studies have shown that fibre-rich foods are a natural appetite suppressant. Because they take up more room in your stomach than other foods, you feel fuller faster. Fibre is slower to digest, so it keeps hunger at bay longer. And most fibre-rich foods take more time to chew (think of muesli vs. a doughnut), so your brain has more time to register that you have had enough to eat – before you have eaten too much.

Antioxidants for arthritis

Findings from the landmark Framingham study (see p189) indicate that the antioxidant vitamins C, E and beta carotene help to prevent the progression of osteoarthritis. Antioxidants help to neutralize free radicals, the chemicals continually formed within cells during normal metabolism, that can damage cartilage and possibly cause inflammation as well.

Fruits and vegetables are the best sources of antioxidants. The following guidelines suggest how you can maximize your antioxidant intake. Eat:

- Red grapes rather than green or white varieties
- Red and yellow onions instead of white
- Cabbage, cauliflower, and broccoli raw or lightly cooked
- Garlic – raw and crushed
- Fresh and frozen – rather than canned – vegetables
- Microwaved – instead of boiled or steamed – vegetables
- The darkest green leafy vegetables
- Pink grapefruit instead of white grapefruit
- Whole fruits rather than juices
- Fresh and frozen juices instead of canned varieties
- The deepest orange carrots, sweet potatoes and pumpkins

- Garnish your cereal with sliced bananas, berries, raisins or other fruit. You need only a quarter cup of dried fruit, half a cup of berries, or one medium banana or other fruit to make a full serving.

- Make an omelette using plenty of vegetables – onions, peppers, tomatoes or any others that appeal to you. Half a cup of chopped vegetables provides you with one serving. For an extra boost, drink tomato or vegetable juice.

The antioxidant impact of fruits and vegetables extends far beyond vitamins C, E and beta carotene. These foods also contain hundreds and perhaps thousands of different phytochemicals (substances found only in plants). Many of them appear to function as antioxidants, and only a small fraction of them have been identified.

▶ Prepare your lunchtime salad using watercress, romaine lettuce or spinach. (Avoid iceberg lettuce, as it is the least nutritious of all vegetable greens.)

▶ Add tomatoes, sliced peppers, shredded carrots or bean sprouts when making sandwiches.

▶ When it's time for a healthy snack, don't settle for sticks of celery or carrots. Expand your snack menu to encompass raw broccoli, cauliflower, green beans and slices of red and green peppers.

▶ Take along raw vegetables as an extra when you are making a packed lunch.

▶ Drink fruit or vegetable juices rather than coffee or tea during work breaks. Buy a pack of small boxes of juice that are easy to carry with you.

Where to find vitamins

Now that you know what antioxidant vitamins can help your arthritis, how can you make sure you get them? Here is a guide to what foods contain which nutrients:

Beta carotene Yellow-orange fruits and vegetables such as apricots, sweet potatoes, pumpkin, carrots, melon, mangoes, pawpaw, peaches and squash, as well as dark green leafy vegetables such as broccoli, spinach, spring greens, parsley and other leafy greens.

Vitamin C Peaches, grapefruit, pawpaw, kiwi fruit, oranges, mangoes, raspberries, pineapples, bananas, strawberries, tomatoes and vegetables such as Brussels sprouts, spring greens, cabbage, asparagus, broccoli, potatoes and red peppers.

Vitamin E Sunflower and safflower oils, sunflower seeds, wheat germ, nuts, avocados, parsnips, whole-grain breads and cereals, spinach, broccoli, asparagus, dried prunes and peanut butter.

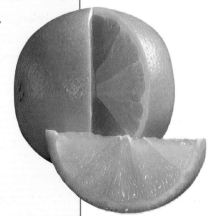

● When you prepare pasta for dinner, remember that a half cup of tomato sauce qualifies as a serving of cooked vegetable.

● Prepare several fruit desserts each week, such as stewed apple, poached pears or that old favourite, jelly with pieces of fruit in it.

● Natural yoghurt is tastier and healthier if you add strawberries, raspberries or sliced apples, bananas, peaches or plums.

caution

To be on the safe side, avoid single-nutrient vitamin D supplements. If you happen to be using a margarine fortified with vitamin D, taking D supplements could actually tip your intake into the danger zone.

Portion sizes: Aim at five servings of vegetables and fruit a day. A single serving of vegetables is ½ cup cooked or raw vegetables, 1 cup leafy raw vegetables or ½ cup cooked pulses. A single serving of fruit is 1 medium apple, ½ grapefruit, banana or orange, 1 melon wedge, 1 small glass (3½fl oz/100ml) pure fruit juice, 6 tbsp (5oz/140g) diced, cooked or canned fruit.

> ● **FACT** You will encourage yourself to eat more fruit if you put it out where you can see it – in a bowl on a worktop or coffee table rather than in a refrigerator.

Dairy foods for healthy bones

The third food group includes the dairy foods – milk, yogurt and cheese – as well as meat, fish, pulses, eggs and nuts. As we progress further up our notional pyramid, the fewer the number of daily servings we recommend. That is because the lower-calorie, more nutrient-rich foods belong in the biggest group.

Dairy products provide most of the calcium in our diets; they also provide proteins for growth and repair, and are important for women in staving off osteoporosis. In addition, they are our main source of vitamin D, which – although not an antioxidant – is crucially important when it comes to osteoarthritis. To limit your fat intake, try to have low-fat or non-fat versions of dairy foods, such as semi-skimmed milk and low-fat yoghurt.

Portion sizes Try to have two to three portions a day; a single portion is ⅓pint (7fl oz) milk or a small pot of yoghurt, 4½oz cottage cheese or fromage frais or 1½oz Cheddar cheese.

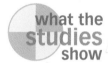

what the studies show

● US researchers at the University of North Carolina at Chapel Hill recently measured levels of 11 antioxidant phytochemicals in the blood of 200 people with OA of the knee and 200 people who did not have the problem. Having higher blood levels of several phytochemicals – beta cryptoxanthine, lutein and lycopene – was associated with a 30 to 40 per cent reduction in the risk of developing OA. These phytochemicals are found in leafy green and brightly coloured vegetables. Tomatoes, for example, contain high levels of lycopene.

◗ **FACT** Always opt for low-fat or non-fat dairy products. Full-fat milk and cheese are high in fat and calories – the main causes of weight gain. Lower-fat varieties provide the same beneficial nutrients as their full-fat counterparts.

The power of protein

Lean meat, poultry, fish, pulses, eggs, nuts and the vegetarian alternatives are your best sources of protein and also supply you with B vitamins, iron and zinc. Obviously, the lower-fat choices in this category are pulses or fish, but there are sensible ways to cut the fat content from meat; choosing leaner cuts of meat, and trimming off the fat before cooking can make the difference between a high-fat and slimmer meal. Remember that with poultry, light meat is lower in fat than dark meat – by about 50 per cent – and the fatty skin should be removed.

Only moderate amounts of protein-rich foods are required in a balanced diet: protein should provide about 11 per cent of your daily calories.

Portion sizes: Eat two to four portions a day. A single portion consists of 2-3oz (55-85g) cooked, lean meat, 4-5oz (115-140g) white or oily fish (not fried), or 5oz (140g) baked beans or 2oz (55g) nuts. (For vegetarians, it is useful to know that 1 egg or 2 tbsp of peanut butter count as 1oz (25g) meat.)

Melting moments

The smallest group of foods contains the fats and sweets that should be eaten sparingly. These foods are very rich in calories but tend to offer fewer of the body-building nutrients other food groups contain. Examples include fat-filled foods such as butter and margarine, and sugar-rich foods such as sweets and soft drinks, or sugar and fat-rich biscuits and cakes. These tempting and calorific foods can pose a major stumbling block to your weight-loss efforts. And don't forget that a lot of foods have hidden sugars – especially processed foods.

Portion sizes Try to have no more than two portions a day, but preferably fewer. A single portion is 3 teaspoons of sugar, a heaped teaspoon of jam or honey, a Danish pastry, 2 biscuits, a small bar of chocolate or half a slice of cake.

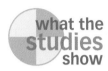

what the studies show

◗ A 1996 US study suggests that vitamin D intake may influence osteoarthritis. Researchers found that people who consumed less than 10mcg a day were about three times more likely to experience a worsening of their knee OA than people who consumed more. At the time, 10mcg was the Recommended Daily Allowance in the USA; the US National Institutes of Health now suggest an adequate daily intake (AI) of 5mcg of vitamin D for people under 50 and 10mcg for over-fifties. In Europe the RDA is 5mcg.

Finding out the fat

Meat, full-fat dairy products, nuts, oils and desserts are responsible for most of the fat in people's diets. If you are overweight, cutting back on the fat in these foods is your first task. Taken gram for gram, fat contains more than twice as many calories as carbohydrates or protein (9 calories in a gram of fat against 4 in a gram of carbohydrate or protein).

To make it even more unfair, researchers now know that not all calories are the same: calories from fat are the worst for weight-conscious consumers, since they are more efficiently stored as fat in the body than are calories from carbohydrates or protein. On top of the extra weight it causes, a diet high in fat – especially the saturated fat found in animal products – harms the body in other ways, such as raising blood cholesterol levels and increasing the likelihood of developing certain cancers.

Although over-consumption of fat is a major cause of weight and health problems, the body does need a certain amount, to provide fat-soluble vitamins and essential fatty-acids. These are required for the development and function of the brain, eyes and nervous system. But the amount actually needed is small – only

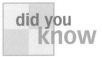
did you know

● Consider using fruit juices or fat-free chicken or beef stock instead of butter or oils when sautéeing vegetables.

A calorie calculator

Here's a shorthand way to tally up the calories you take in when eating servings from the food groups:

Food Group	One serving provides about
Grains	80 calories
Vegetables	25 calories
Fruit	60-80 calories
Meat, poultry, fish, pulses, eggs and nuts	150-250 calories
Milk, yoghurt and cheese	150-200 calories

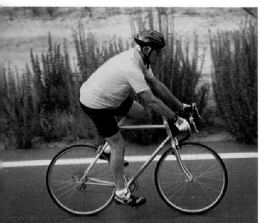

about 1oz (25g) a day – much less than we regularly consume in an average Western diet. The best sources of essential fatty acids are natural fish oils and pure vegetable oils. But when vegetable oils are hardened (hydrogenated) to make margarine and reduced fat spreads, they can be changed into trans fats, which are considered as unhealthy as saturated fats. In the UK it is currently recommended that no more than 33 per cent of our daily calorie intake should come from fats and, of these, no more than 10 per cent from saturated fats and 2 per cent from trans fats.

Fortunately, by shopping wisely, you can significantly reduce the amount of fat – and the percentage of calories from fat – in your diet. The table below illustrates some major differences in fat among foods that otherwise are quite similar. To single out one example: pretzels and potato crisps are both salty snacks, but there is a dramatic difference: 1oz of potato crisps contains 11 times more total fat than 1oz of pretzel twists.

Fats in foods

Food		Total fat in grams	Calories	% of calories from fat
Tuna	Chunk light in brine or water, 3oz (85g), undrained	1.0	89	10
	Chunk light in vegetable oil, 3oz (85g), undrained	17.6	254	62
Chicken	Roasted light meat, no skin, 3½oz (100g)	4.5	171	24
	Fried, battered, light meat, with skin, 3½oz	15.3	274	50
Meat	Sirloin steak, lean only, grilled, 3oz (85g)	7.7	180	39
	Sirloin steak, lean and fat, grilled, 3oz (85g)	15.7	240	59
Milk	Skimmed milk, 8fl oz (225ml)	0.4	86	4
	Whole milk, 8fl oz (225ml)	8.1	150	49
Ice cream	Vanilla-flavoured low-fat frozen dessert, 4fl oz (125ml)	0.4	70	5
	Vanilla ice cream, 4fl oz (125ml)	17.9	260	62
Snacks	Pretzel twists, 1oz (25g)	0.9	110	7
	Potato crisps, 1oz (25g)	11.7	160	66

Reading the fine print

Knowing your way around the nutritional analysis labels found on most food packaging can save calories and fat.

Here are some indications of what the fine print says – and what the UK Food Standards Agency recommends it should mean:

◗ Fat-free: less than 0.15g of fat in 100g of product

◗ Low-fat: 3g of fat or less in 100g of product

◗ Reduced fat: at least 25 per cent less fat than its full-fat equivalent

◗ Light or lite: there is no legal definition, so check the fat and calorie content carefully on these products.

Beware A product that claims to be 'light' may contain the same amount of fat and calories as a standard version of another brand. Try to compare products that claim to be fat-reduced in any way, with normal versions of the product.

Portion sizes Try to keep your fat intake to between one and five portions a day. A portion can be 1 teaspoon (5ml) of butter or margarine, 2 teaspoons of low-fat spread, 1 teaspoon of cooking oil, 1 tablespoon of mayonnaise or salad dressing, 1 tablespoon of cream or a single-serving packet of crisps.

◗ **FACT** Regular exercise can be extremely effective in weight control. In fact, study after study shows that dieting alone can help people lose weight – but that exercise is needed to keep it off.

Make changes slowly

Changing something as basic as what you eat – tofu instead of steak, say – can be very difficult. You are most likely to succeed over the long term if you proceed gradually. Here are some tips for making modest changes that, over time, can really add up:

▶ If you take whole milk in your coffee, try switching to semi-skimmed milk (1.7g of fat in 100ml) for a few weeks, then to skimmed milk (0.1g of fat in 100ml).

▶ Eat more slowly. By doing so, you will find that you start to feel satisfied with smaller portions.

▶ Don't let meat, chicken or fish dominate your plate – make vegetables the largest serving, instead.

▶ Cut the amount of meat in a recipe by half; use only lean meats, and fill in the lost bulk with shredded vegetables, pulses, pasta, grains or other low-fat ingredients.

▶ Brighten meals with variety. When you go shopping, buy a fruit or vegetable that you've never tried before.

▶ When you leave for work or on a day's outing, make a packed lunch to avoid buying fat-filled fast food.

Watch those portions

Nutrition experts all seem to agree: we have an exaggerated idea of what size a serving should be. Restaurants in particular are to blame for making more seem better, in the minds of consumers.

▶ **FACT** One sure way to sabotage a diet, experts agree, is to rule out certain foods entirely. Rather than consider any food forbidden, you should instead eat small portions of it fairly regularly. For example, instead of denying yourself your weekly whole deep-pan pizza, share it and have just one or two slices instead.

The clear trend in the UK has been toward consuming larger food portions (see *Size does matter*, right), especially of foods rich in fat and sugar. The result, not surprisingly, has been an unbalanced diet. At the same time, our

Size does matter

This chart (with approximate calorie values) shows the larger amounts now often offered as single portions:

Food	Recommended portion	Typical portion 1977	Large portion 2003
Cola drink	—	12fl oz/350ml (120 kcal)	44fl oz/1125ml (412 kcal)
French fries	10 (160 kcal)	About 30 (475 kcal)	About 50 (790 kcal)
Hamburger	2-3oz/55-85g (240 kcal)	3-4oz/85-115g (330 kcal)	6oz/175g (650 kcal)
Steak	2-3oz/85g (170 kcal)	12oz/350g (690 kcal)	1lb/450-550g (1,260 kcal)
Yoghurt	4oz/115g (100 kcal)	6oz/175g (150 kcal)	8oz/225g (200 kcal)
Baked potato	3-4oz/85-115g (100 kcal)	5-7oz/140-200g (180 kcal)	1lb/450g (420 kcal)
Mars bar	—	2¼oz/65g (294 kcal)	3½oz/100g (452 kcal)
Crisps	—	1oz/25g (90 kcal)	2oz/50g (180 kcal)

collective waistline is expanding as a nation as more people become overweight or obese, suggesting an increasing need to control portion sizes if we are to win the battle of the bulge.

This distorted notion of serving size not only piles on the calories but also gives many people the mistaken idea that eating the recommended five servings of fruit and vegetables a day is impossible. But actually, one serving of fruit is just one medium-sized piece of fresh fruit or about 6 tbsp (5oz/140g) of stewed or canned fruit.

Can you eat yourself better?

The idea that some foods can worsen arthritis, while others may ease its symptoms, is intriguing and controversial. Until recently, most experts were fairly sceptical about diet therapy's role.

Studies over the past few years have shown that some dietary interventions may be of some use, particularly for patients with inflammatory forms of arthritis such as rheumatoid arthritis.

Can you control what you eat?

Ideally, you'll want a diet that follows roughly the recommendations we have made. Keeping a food diary will give you feedback on whether your diet provides the proper number of servings of each food type and whether you're getting enough variety in your food.

For each meal, fill in the number of servings of each food group. Then, at the end of the day, count up the totals for each group. Don't get discouraged if you fall short of the ideal: breaking the habits of many years is seldom done overnight.

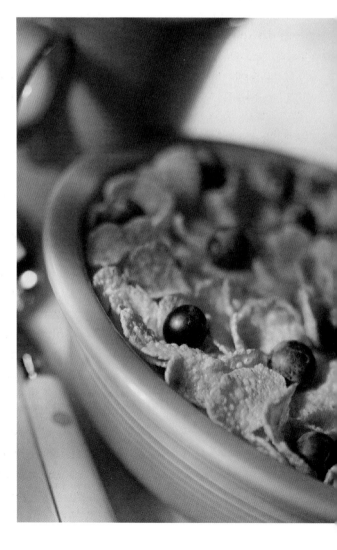

Breakfast   **Number of servings**

Bread

Vegetable

Fruit

Dairy

Meat

Lunch

Bread

Vegetable

Fruit

Dairy

Meat

Dinner

Bread

Vegetable

Fruit

Dairy

Meat

Totals for the day

Bread group servings

Vegetable group servings

Fruit group servings

Dairy group servings

Meat group servings

Below is an overview of specific diets that have been used to treat arthritis – and what the evidence reveals about their effects. It is important to remember, however, that each person's arthritis is different and there is no cure-all.

Elimination or avoidance diets

These are based on the idea that certain foods are the aggressors when it comes to arthritis. Proponents claim that by taking the offending foods out of their diets, people with arthritis will find significant improvements in their symptoms.

The anti-nightshade diet In the USA, one the best-known avoidance diets is based on the idea that members of the 'nightshade' family of foods (tomatoes, potatoes, peppers and aubergine) contain chemicals that not only promote inflammation but also increase pain and interfere with the repair of damaged joints.

The 'nightshade theory' was proposed by a horticulturist who knew that tomatoes and other nightshades were once considered poisonous, and noticed that they seemed to worsen his arthritis. He carried out an uncontrolled study in which more than 5,000 arthritis patients were asked to avoid nightshade foods for seven years; nearly three-quarters of the patients said their pain and disability gradually decreased with the diet.

The bottom line The nightshade-free diet has never been studied in a scientifically rigorous way, though it has been reported that a few patients have improved after nightshade foods were eliminated from their diets. It can't hurt to try the diet (provided you make no radical dietary changes that interfere with balanced nutrition), but don't expect much from it.

The Dong diet Named after Collin Dong, the physician who devised it for his own arthritis, this regime is modelled on a centuries-old Chinese diet and imposes much broader food restrictions than the anti-nightshade diet. Arthritis patients are urged to eat vegetables (except tomatoes) but to eliminate red meat, fruit, dairy foods, herbs, alcohol, soft drinks and all additives and preservatives. In a study published in 1983, some arthritis patients were placed on the Dong diet while others followed a more varied diet. No significant differences were noted; about half the people in each group reported feeling better.

The bottom line No scientific evidence supports the Dong diet, which could actually harm people with arthritis; the diet excludes fruit, which provides antioxidants and other nutrients

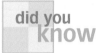
did you know

Nightshades come from the plant genus *Solanum* and include more than 1,700 herbs, shrubs and trees, including eggplant, bell peppers, potatoes, and tomatoes. Although there are many claims that removing nightshades from the diet will cure arthritis, no scientific proof has yet been offered.

Eliminate the negative?

If you suspect that a particular food such as tomatoes makes your arthritis worse, it can't hurt to eliminate that food from your diet and then wait for a couple of weeks to see if you feel better. A more scientifically rigorous – but more drastic – approach is dietary elimination therapy, which should be done only under a doctor's supervision.

This therapy begins with a food elimination phase, designed to clear the system of all possible food culprits. This phase may require a total water-fast lasting for a week, or a less extreme, more nourishing diet consisting perhaps of fish, pears, carrots, water and other foods considered safe to eat. If your symptoms do disappear during the elimination phase, foods are then carefully reintroduced, one at a time, to see which are actually causing the problem.

that are important for the health of joints; and it bans dairy products, the main dietary source of the calcium and vitamin D needed to maintain bones and assist in cartilage formation.

Anti-allergic diets: causing a reaction?

Many arthritis patients become convinced that some foods – particularly milk products, corn and cereals – do more than just aggravate their arthritis; they believe they can actually trigger symptoms in a matter of minutes, such as people with asthma may start coughing after inhaling pollen or other substances to which they're allergic.

Some people do have genuine food allergies, in which a food protein prompts the immune system to produce antibodies against that protein, which is known as an antigen. Antibody combines with antigen to form antigen-antibody 'complexes'. Proponents of the allergy-arthritis notion contend that these antigen-antibody complexes could conceivably irritate the joints or even attack the joints' synovial lining. Experts now believe that food sensitivities such as allergies may be involved in some cases of rheumatoid and other types of inflammatory arthritis.

But the actual proportion of patients affected appears to be quite small – perhaps 5 per cent or fewer. Consider the results of one carefully conducted study that involved 159 patients with rheumatoid arthritis, 52 of whom claimed that food aggravated their symptoms; actual testing of all the patients failed to detect a single case of food intolerance.

Diets that put out the fire

Inflammation is the body's response to tissue damage or to overuse of a diseased joint. Researchers have found that fatty acids may beneficially alter the inflammation response in certain types of arthritis, as can certain chemicals found in teas.

Fishing for relief

Studies of the Inuit people of Greenland led to interest in the anti-arthritic properties of fish. Although they lived mainly on fatty fish, these people were found to have a remarkably low level of heart disease – and of rheumatoid arthritis as well. The beneficial effects of these cold-water fish were attributed to their fat, specifically the omega-3 fatty acids that are plentiful in fish oil.

Researchers now know that eating fish can help to reduce inflammation in several ways. For example, a diet high in fish changes the lipids that make up cell membranes in the body, and this change reduces the level of inflammatory chemicals called cytokines.

Several studies have shown fish-oil supplements may help to ease symptoms in patients with rheumatoid arthritis, for whom inflammation is a major problem. And one recent UK study (see page 187) has shown that cod-liver oil can slow and may reverse the destruction of joint cartilage that occurs in osteoarthritis.

caution

Too much fish or fish oil can interfere with your blood's ability to clot. An excessive intake of fish oil can lead to overdoses of vitamins A and D (especially if you're getting them in your vitamin supplements or through fortified margarine), which can be toxic.

Even if fish or fish-oil supplements don't help to ease your arthritis symptoms, eating more fish makes a lot of sense. Studies show that people who eat fish regularly can gain some important health benefits.

A major study of American men, over a six to eight-year period, found that those consuming the most fish were about 40 per cent less likely to die from a heart attack or a stroke caused by a clot than men who ate the least amount of fish. In addition, researchers have found that omega-3 fatty acids – the kind plentiful in fatty fish – are important nutrients for vision, for nerve and immune function, and possibly for protection against some types of cancer.

In the UK, a study of Sikh men and women, who ate very little oily fish, found that after a moderate intake of oily fish over a 12 week period, the levels of beneficial fatty acids in their bodies had increased to the levels of people who did eat fish regularly.

> ● **FACT** Eicosapentaenoic acid (EPA), best known of the omega-3 fatty acids, is found in marine plants and fish. EPA is actually made by algae, plankton and seaweed, which are then eaten by certain fish.

Fat content of selected oily fish

Food (3oz/85g)	Omega-3 fatty acids (g)	Saturated fat (g)	Total fat (g)	Calories
Salmon	1.9	1.1	6.9	155
Herring	1.8	2.2	9.8	172
Whitefish	1.6	1.0	6.4	146
Tuna (fresh)	1.3	1.4	5.3	156
Sardines, canned, in oil	1.3	1.3	9.7	177
Mackerel	1.1	3.6	15.2	223
Rainbow trout	1.0	1.4	5.0	128

The bottom line All fish contain some omega-3 fatty acids. But to maximize your intake, choose oily cold-water fish such as salmon, tuna and mackerel (see the table on page 222). Eating cold-water fish two or three times a week should help your overall health and could be of some help to your arthritis.

Sip your arthritis symptoms away

If you have arthritis or simply want to improve your general health, put the kettle on and have a cup of tea; that old British cure for all crises does have scientific backing. Researchers have long known that tea is rich in flavonoids, a class of phyto-chemicals known for its antioxidant abilities. Some studies have shown that regular tea drinkers are up to 50 per cent less likely to develop certain types of cancer compared with non-tea drinkers, while other studies have found that regular tea drinkers have a lower risk of stroke and heart disease. And as noted earlier in this chapter, evidence suggests that diets rich in antioxidants can help to keep osteoarthritis from worsening.

The green light to green tea Both black and green teas are good sources of flavonoids, but now there is reason to believe that green tea may be useful against rheumatoid arthritis, thanks to a different class of phytochemicals known as polyphenols, present in large amounts. Green tea also contains compounds called catechins, which are associated with alleviating several conditions such as stroke, heart disease and even cancer. Dr. David Buttle at Sheffield University in the UK, has found that catechins in green tea (EGCG and ECG) can block the enzyme that destroys cartilage. As the destruction of cartilage is one of the major factors in osteoarthritis, Dr. Buttle believes that drinking green tea could play a part in preventing the development of OA. He says that if you have fairly severe joint damage, it may be too late to do anything about it, but if you drink green tea throughout your life, it may be beneficial and prevent disease.

The bottom line Try drinking three or four cups of green tea daily, without milk, to see if it reduces inflammation. Note: Green tea does contain caffeine (about 40mg a cup), so to compensate, you may want to cut back on other sources of caffeine such as coffee.

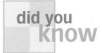

did you **know**

▶ Letting green tea infuse for more than 5 minutes can cause the beneficial substances to lose their potency. Use 1 teaspoon of green tea leaves in each cup of very hot (not boiling) water.

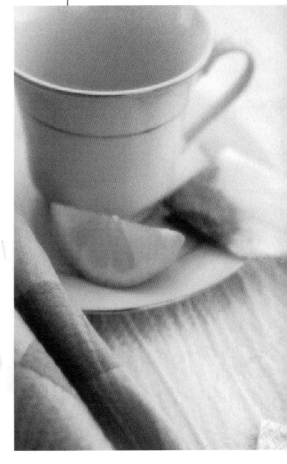

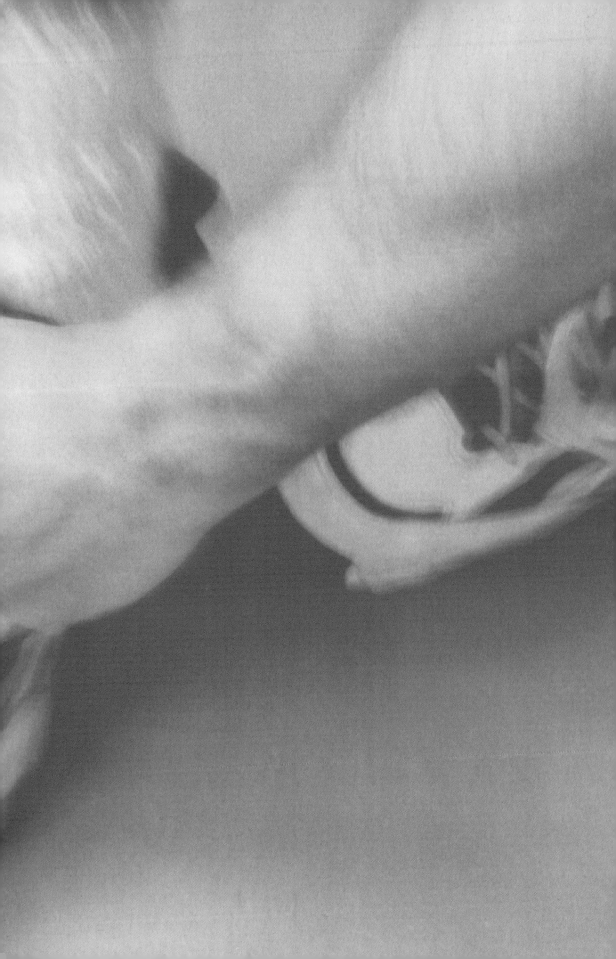

8

Get moving

The human body is built to move. That might seem painfully contradictory to an arthritis patient, but exercise is indeed medicine in motion: it can help to prevent osteoarthritis, and it can certainly help those already living with the condition.

Resisting the siren call of the armchair

Exercising an arthritic joint seems masochistic; when a joint is aching, no one in their right mind would think that swimming, cycling or walking would make it better. But it does. Inactivity leads to the wasting away of muscle, which can increase the strain on joints – and that causes even more pain.

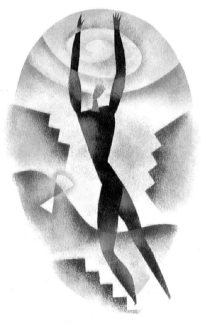

EXERCISE is one of the pillars of the take-charge philosophy. It is not only vital for weight loss – vital for anyone with arthritis – but also essential to the health of your joints.

Until a few years ago, doctors endorsed their patients' tendency towards inactivity by advising them to stay off their feet. They assumed that osteoarthritis was an inevitable part of ageing and that exercise just made things worse by speeding up cartilage destruction. As for patients with rheumatoid arthritis, doctors believed that joint-jolting exercise would do nothing but trigger inflammation and flare-ups.

The healing power of movement They were so wrong. Science, fortunately, has had the last word on the subject, proving that exercise is good medicine for arthritis sufferers. Study after study has shown that moderate activity does not damage joints or worsen arthritis pain. In fact, regular exercise is one of the best therapies for relieving joint pain and also improves many other health problems common to arthritis patients.

Activity's wide range of benefits

Arthritis can have a physically damaging effect – and not just on the joints; studies show that many people with arthritis are in general poor health, especially when it comes to risk factors for heart disease.

Compared with people of the same age, who do not suffer from arthritis, people who have arthritis tend to be much heavier and have higher blood pressure, lower levels of HDL cholesterol (the 'good' form that prevents heart disease), and higher blood sugar levels (indicating possible diabetes). And the reason for most of this is inactivity – which was recently declared a major heart-disease risk factor.

FACT Strong, well-toned muscles, tendons and ligaments can bear the brunt of the force on our joints as we move. In fact, most of the load that the joints bear can be transferred to these supporting structures, taking some of the load off the cartilage.

Exercise offers numerous health benefits to people no matter what their age or their physical condition, but it can be especially valuable for people with arthritis. Regular activity can relieve pain and stiffness as effectively as NSAIDs and other drugs – while offering two crucial additional advantages:

● Drugs – especially the pain-relieving NSAIDs – can cause serious and potentially fatal side effects, while exercise rarely causes significant problems.

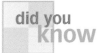
did you know

● One in every eight people over the age of 65 has to limit his or her activity in some way as a result of arthritis.

Small moves, big gains

Scientific evidence shows that doing moderate exercise regularly will yield the following benefits:

● Reduced risk of death from all causes

● Reduced risk of developing heart disease

● Reduced risk of high blood pressure (and lowered blood pressure in people who are already hypertensive)

● Help in weight loss and weight management

● Reduced risk of several types of cancer, including colon, prostate and, possibly, breast cancer

● Reduced risk of stroke

● Improved blood glucose control in people with Type 2 (adult-onset) diabetes and less risk of diabetes-related complications

● Reduced anxiety and depression

● Improved quality of sleep

> Drugs and exercise can both relieve symptoms, but exercise does something that no drug can do: modifies the course of arthritis by making joints healthier – stopping osteoarthritis from worsening and perhaps even preventing the disease from occurring.

Besides relieving pain and stiffness, the right combination of exercises can help to strengthen and stabilize arthritic joints and prevent them from becoming deformed. Equally important, exercise can reduce mental stress that can exacerbate physical pain. And if you need further motivation to get moving, staying active can lower your risk of diabetes, hypertension, heart disease and several types of cancer; provide relief from insomnia and depression; and improve immunity and a sense of well-being.

did you know

> When muscles are immobilized – through complete bed rest, for example – they can lose 3 per cent of their strength each day.

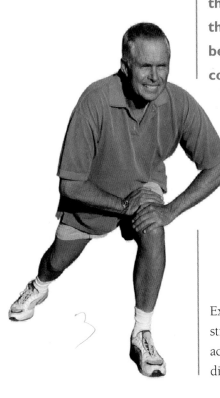

Exercise and joints: working together

The well-known fitness adage 'Use it or lose it' certainly applies to your joints. Unless you put them through their paces with regular activity, they lose their strength and resilience and become weaker, stiffer, more painful and constricted. That's because exercise (or the lack of it) affects the health of all parts of a joint, including the bones and the all-important cartilage that covers the ends of them.

> **FACT** Bones are dynamic, not static, constantly changing in response to the demands placed on them. Bones are like muscles, growing thicker and stronger in response to a heavier work load.

Experts recommend three types of exercise for arthritis sufferers: stretching to increase range-of-motion; aerobic or weight-bearing activities like walking; and strength training. Each works in a different but important way to strengthen and improve joints.

> ## How often should you exercise?
>
> ● Try to do stretching (range-of-motion) exercises every day or at least every other day.
>
> ● Strengthening exercises should be done every other day, so that muscles can rest between workouts.
>
> ● Try to do aerobic exercises or walk for 20 to 30 minutes three times a week.

Be flexible

The joint's range of motion – how fully and easily you can bend your knees to pick up a pencil or your grandchild, for example – depends on the flexibility of the muscles, tendons and ligaments that surround and protect it.

When pain and stiffness discourage people from moving their joints, the inactivity causes these surrounding tissues to contract, which further limits the joint's movement. Stretching exercises are vital for flexible muscles, tendons and ligaments, so that the range of movement can be maintained and even enhanced.

Strengthen the joint's support

The bones of a joint do not operate in isolation. Their ability to move depends on the muscles and tendons that pull on them. Exercises aimed at strengthening muscles and tendons can ease movement and help the joints to move with less pain. Bulking up the muscle mass around a joint also helps to protect the joint in the event of a fall or any other physical assault on the area.

We all tend to lose muscle mass as we get older, a reality which unfortunately exacts a double penalty on older arthritis sufferers; not only do they lose muscle mass quite naturally as they age but they also lose it because of the inactivity that is so often a consequence of their painful condition.

This is why muscle-strengthening exercises are valuable for all older people, but especially for those with arthritis.

> 'Exercise is the best thing you can do if you have arthritis, and keeping as active and fit as you can will only do you good and will not damage the joints.'
>
> – Dr. Mike Hurley, physiotherapist, Dulwich Hospital, King's Healthcare Trust, London

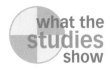

> Recent studies suggest that defects in the bone just beneath a joint's cartilage may play a role in causing osteoarthritis. Weight-bearing exercise is known to stimulate bone growth – it helps to ward off the bone-thinning disorder osteoporosis, for example – and its effect on bone may protect against osteoarthritis, too.

Caring for your cartilage

Smooth movement within a joint depends on the health of its cartilage. (It is the wearing away of cartilage where the bones come together that results in the pain and stiffness of OA.) To maximize the health of a joint and its cartilage, the joint must not only move regularly but must actually undergo 'repetitive joint loading' – the stress exerted by aerobic, weight-bearing exercises such as walking or jogging.

> **FACT** For every year that you have been out of shape, you need a month or more to get back into shape.

A brief anatomy lesson Remember that cartilage is not solid like bone, but supple and flexible – contracting and expanding like a sponge each time weight is applied to it. The cartilage in your knee, for example, compresses slightly each time you take a step and then, as you step onto your other foot, it expands to return to its resting shape.

The spongy cartilage is filled with and surrounded by synovial fluid, which is soaked up and then wrung out with each step. This soak-and-squeeze action lubricates the cartilage, preventing it from drying out and becoming stiff. But perhaps even more important, this repetitive stress also stimulates cartilage growth and repair.

Unlike most tissues, cartilage doesn't have blood vessels that can supply its nourishment. Instead, cartilage must get nutrients from the synovial fluid that bathes it. Only through the repetitive stress from weight-bearing activities can chondrocytes (the cartilage-making cells) receive the nutrients that make them produce more cartilage. If you already have arthritis, weight-bearing exercise can help to maintain your remaining cartilage and help to stop the disease in its tracks. Also, maintaining cartilage health through regular weight-bearing exercise may actually help to prevent osteoarthritis from occurring in the first place.

In the absence of a cure, exercise is arguably the best available therapy for arthritis of all kinds. The less active you have been until now, the more dramatic the benefits are likely to be.

Small steps make a big difference

Generally, as people get older, in the UK and elsewhere, they tend to do less and less exercise. In a way, this exercise antipathy is understandable: intense exercise and macho slogans such as 'No pain, no gain' are enough to discourage anyone from putting on a pair of trainers and going out. Fortunately, the best exercise slogan today is actually a very old one: 'All things in moderation'.

Lifestyle fitness The value of moderate exercise is endorsed by the Health Development Agency, which says there is evidence that getting enough exercise is an important contributor to overall health and well-being – and you don't have to go to the gym to achieve this. Their advice is to do 30 minutes of moderate activity, on at least five days a week. This could include activities such as walking, cycling, gardening or even cleaning the house. Their figures show that only 25 per cent of women and 37 per cent of men in the UK meet this target.

> **FACT** On days when you really don't feel motivated, plan to exercise for just 5 minutes. If you still don't feel like exercising after this length of time, stop. Most of the time, however, you'll start feeling invigorated and you will want to continue.

A simple change in your lifestyle, such as walking up stairs, rather than taking the lift or escalator, is just one example of how to increase your daily activity. Try to set aside some time to do things that you enjoy or have enjoyed in the past – such as dancing, going for walks, cycling or swimming.

If you enjoy doing the activity you are more likely to stick to it and do it more often. You could get off the bus one stop earlier and walk the extra distance, or go for a walk at lunchtime. Cutting down on the time you spend in front of the television or computer will also help.

did you know

You don't have to do all your exercising in one long session. You'll gain nearly the same health benefits by breaking it up into shorter segments throughout the day, whenever you have some spare time.

This 'exercise prescription' is amply supported by research showing that moderate activity offers many of the same health benefits previously associated with full-throttle exercise.

The good news about moderate exercise couldn't come at a better time for people with arthritis. Studies have shown that it is safe for virtually all arthritis patients to engage in moderate exercise – and extremely useful as well: low-impact aerobics, swimming, dancing, walking and cycling are all examples of moderate exercise that can ease joint pain and stiffness, while also improving your overall health.

The essence of taking charge

The best way to incorporate exercise into your daily routine is to make it a key aspect of your take-charge plan. Most arthritis patients can find some form of exercise that is appropriate – and even fun – for them. And of all possible treatment approaches, exercise may be the one most likely to lead to self-empowerment.

By now, you know how important it is for arthritis patients to embrace the belief that they can control their own destiny. In study after study, self-empowered patients have proved most successful in overcoming their symptoms and leading richer, fuller lives. Choose a long-term goal and then reach it through a succession of short-term goals – it's tailor-made for exercise.

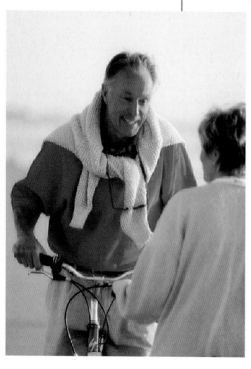

Exercise builds confidence Studies have already shown that exercise gives people confidence that they can meet the physical challenges of life – the essence of self-empowerment.

Actions can be specified A key element in taking charge of arthritis is your take-charge plan (see page 106), in which you list the actions you hope to achieve each week. Exercise is ideal for your take-charge plan, as you can express it as a number of repetitions (12 leg lifts, for example), a distance ('walk 1 mile'), a length of time ('do stretching exercises for 10 minutes') or perhaps even specify its intensity ('walk 10 minutes on a treadmill set at 3.5 miles an hour').

Keeping score is easy. You know whether you've met your target goal of 'two sets of 12 leg lifts on Monday, Wednesday and Friday'. Meeting your score each day will encourage you.

You can make adjustments If doing 12 leg lifts proves too difficult, reduce your repetitions to ten. It is never good to do more than you feel capable of, and straining yourself will not benefit you in the long term.

It is easy to build on your success The take-charge plan is based on gradual progress – achieving small successes each week until you finally achieve a goal that may once have seemed out of your reach. A well-planned exercise programme will follow the same pattern, with requirements becoming slightly more strenuous from week to week.

Ask the experts

For most people, exercise is a simple proposition: put on a pair of trainers or a swimsuit, start exercising and sweat. But for arthritis patients who may have damaged a joint, strained the supporting ligaments or tendons, or have muscle imbalances, consulting your doctor and possibly a physiotherapist may be a better first move.

Physiotherapists are exercise specialists who can work with you to create a programme of stretching, strengthening and aerobic exercises that is tailored to your needs and abilities. You may be in particular need of that kind of advice if your arthritis is severe or if you stopped exercising a long time ago.

Getting physical A physiotherapist will assess your aerobic capacity, your sense of balance, the flexibility of all your joints and your muscular strength. Then the therapist will develop a programme targeted at areas where you need help – quadriceps-strengthening exercises for knee pain, for example, or swimming to improve aerobic capacity and overall flexibility. Ideally, the choices will include activities you enjoy, so you'll be motivated to stick with the programme for years to come.

A course of physiotherapy generally lasts just a few weeks, although some people may benefit from longer-term care. Therapy sessions usually last less than an hour and may range in frequency from once a week to every day.

The best way to find a physiotherapist is to ask your doctor for a referral to a chartered physiotherapist. Physiotherapists work in hospitals, clinics, health clubs, sport injury clinics and nursing homes. Some of them even make house calls. Make sure your physiotherapist is fully aware of your medical condition – this will ensure that your programme is absolutely right for you.

did you know

▶ If pain is your excuse to skip exercise, try a dose of moist heat first. Applying moist heat packs, taking tolerably hot baths or showers, soaking in a hot tub, or swimming in a well-heated pool can help you to get moving.

Exercise incentives to keep you moving

▶ Get a workout partner. If someone is depending on you for exercise, you will be more likely to get up and out instead of snoozing by the fire.

▶ Log it. Placing a red X on a calendar on the days you exercise, or writing about specifics of a workout in a notebook, can turn exercise into a major part of your life.

▶ Buy yourself a gadget or fashionable accessory. A new heart-rate monitor, a fancy leotard or a colourful pair of trainers can be all it takes to get you out and about.

▶ Music makes it better. Studies show that people who read or watch television while they exercise, may perform with less power and intensity, but the music has been found to stimulate the feel-good chemicals of the brain, called endorphins, which makes it all the more enjoyable.

▶ Get competitive. Training for an event or competition can prevent boredom.

▶ Become a morning person. Exercise first thing in the morning and your exercise will be over and done with, no matter how busy your day becomes.

▶ Combine your workout with work. Cycle or walk to work or find ways to do some exercise in your lunch hour.

▶ Don't force it. On your 'down' days, do just a few minutes of exercise rather than neglecting it completely.

Stretching it: unlocking the joints

Of the three types of exercise recommended for arthritis, stretching is the one you should probably do every day. It is the least likely of the three types to cause injury or to aggravate your condition – this is one of the reasons that some stretching exercises may be recommended even during arthritis flare-ups.

Don't let stiffness take over Stretching addresses a problem that affects everyone, whether they have arthritis or not: the tendency for muscles, ligaments, tendons and joints to stiffen with age. Without regular stretching exercises, the average adult's flexibility declines by roughly 5 per cent a decade.

Adding arthritis to the mix makes things considerably worse, since people with the condition are even less likely than others to maintain supple joints. The good news is that inflexible joints can be unlocked – and a conscientious stretching programme can help to erase decades'-worth of accumulated joint tightness.

> **◆ FACT** Stretching exercises to reduce pain are considered a mainstay of treatment for fibromyalgia, a disease that mainly affects women and is characterized by chronic, generalized musculoskeletal pain.

Why it works The concept behind stretching (also known as range-of-motion exercises) is simple: when a muscle is pulled slightly beyond its normal length, it gradually adapts to its longer length and increases a joint's range of motion. This improved range accounts for most of the benefits of stretching – being able to tie your shoes, work in the garden or turn your head while reversing your car, to watch the space behind you.

The basics of stretching

Stretching can be done in several different ways, but there is one technique – static stretching – which is probably safest and is also simple and effective. Static stretching involves easing into a stretch to the point where you begin to feel mild discomfort – never farther – and then holding that maximum position for 10 to 30 seconds. Research has shown that holding a stretch longer than that provides no extra benefits – and that briefer stretches probably won't do you any good.

Water is an ideal place to stretch, since it supports your limbs and helps to minimize the stress on them as you put them through their range of motion. Exercising in warm water – between 83°F (28°C) and 90°F (34°C) is especially useful, as warmth helps to relax muscles and decrease joint pain.

now and then

◆ In 1998, the American College of Sports Medicine expanded the traditional goals of exercise – developing aerobic fitness and muscle strength – to include a third key goal: flexibility. The college urged all Americans to add stretching to their regular exercise programmes, based on the 'growing evidence of its multiple benefits'.

caution

Avoid what is known as 'bounce' stretching – repeated, brief, forceful stretches. They can actually cause damage and increase stiffness.

Stretching do's and don'ts

▶ Your body needs to be prepared for stretching. Never stretch a cold muscle; always warm up first. Do your stretching at the end of your exercise routine, or warm up your muscles with a slow walk or with a 5-10 minute session on the treadmill – then stretch.

▶ For most stretches it is best to be down on the floor so that you can relax your body, especially the area that you are stretching. If you don't relax the area you are stretching, your muscles will tighten slightly and you won't make much progress.

▶ Don't hold your breath while stretching. Your muscles need the oxygen. Exhale as you try to stretch, breathe in, then exhale again as you try to stretch farther.

▶ Stop if you feel any pain. Pain does not, in fact, indicate gain, but rather that you are damaging tissues. You should feel the stretch, but it should not hurt.

▶ The correct technique is important. Don't cheat when you stretch by contorting your body or using other joints to compensate for inflexibility. More flexibility can be acquired with practice.

▶ If you feel any unusual pains or feel sick in any way, stop – and consult your doctor before doing anything more.

Strength training: getting muscle from metal

You may well think that strength training is only for glamorous young people in leotards, heaving around barbells that exceed their own body weight. So you may be surprised to learn that older people are the ones who should be going to the gym. The reason? The older people get, the faster they lose muscle strength.

Believe it or not, between the ages of 20 and 50, muscle strength in the average adult dips by only about 10 to 20 per cent. But over the next two decades, remaining strength falls by an extra 25 to 30 per cent – and drops even faster after that. Inactivity accounts for much of this muscle loss, so it stands to reason that older people with arthritis become even weaker than other people their age.

> ❍ **FACT** Holding your breath when strength training can elevate blood pressure to dangerous levels. Olympic weightlifters have been known to drive their blood pressure to as high as 480/320mmHg. Instead, breathe out while lifting the weight and breathe in while lowering it.

Losing more than muscle As your muscles slowly fade, it can have serious consequences for your daily life. Many older people have some difficulty performing everyday tasks such as carrying the laundry upstairs, opening windows or simply getting out of a chair. Muscle loss also weakens the bones, which need stimulation from the muscles to stay strong. And, of course, the inactivity brought on by arthritis weakens the muscles around joints, limiting a person's ability to move and eventually impairing balance.

However, there is a silver lining: strength training can almost entirely reverse the muscle loss that has occurred over decades. One study, for example, found that 70-year-old men who had engaged in strength training since middle age were just as strong, on average, as 28-year-olds who did no strength training. Furthermore, it appears that the older people get, the greater is their gain, in proportion, from a programme of strength training.

One study found that frail individuals in their 80s and 90s were able to double or even triple their leg strength after strength training for just two months, enabling some of them to start walking without assistance.

More muscle, less pain Strength training has also produced impressive results in studies involving arthritis patients, particularly those with OA of the knee. Almost invariably, the inactivity brought on by OA of the knee causes weakening of the quadriceps muscle, the large muscle at the front of the thigh that

Women who worry that strength training may make them look too bulky and muscular can relax. It won't happen, no matter how hard you train, since women have very little testosterone, the hormone that fuels muscle growth. Yet women can build muscle strength as rapidly as men, even after their muscles have attained peak size.

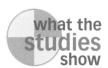

Performed properly, strength training does more than build muscle. Studies show that it also reduces levels of artery-clogging LDL cholesterol and may actually help to reduce blood pressure.

runs from the knee to the hip. Exercises that strengthen the quadriceps muscle can produce striking improvements, greatly easing pain and allowing much more movement of the knee joint.

What's more, strength training helps you to stay slim because the muscle it builds burns calories faster than fat does, even while you're resting. In general, a strength-training session will use up calories as fast as walking does.

In south London, a group of 450 people aged over 50, with OA of the knee are taking part in a new five-year research project to investigate the effectiveness of a rehabilitation programme made up of exercising leg muscles, self-help advice and coping strategies. This will be compared with the typical approach of NSAID prescription. All the patients will take part in exercise sessions – including strength, balance and co-ordination on a bicycle or other simple equipment. If the programme is successful, the programme could become available to NHS patients with OA of the knee, all over the country.

At the end of this chapter, we describe several exercises that can help you to strengthen your quadriceps muscle if OA of the knee is your problem.

Building muscle power

Strength training involves exerting your muscles against resistance – which can be provided by dumbbells, barbells, weight machines, elastic bands or even your own body weight. Engaging in at least two muscle-strengthening sessions a week will build muscle – and even just one weekly session will slow muscle loss and possibly stop it entirely. The sessions need not be time-consuming; you can obtain substantial benefits from as few as four to six exercises that work the major muscles in the arms, shoulders, chest, back and legs.

Performing one set of eight to 12 repetitions of a particular strength-training exercise should improve muscle strength and endurance. Interestingly, for the average person, doing multiple sets provides no additional benefits (at least for the first six months) while increasing the risk of injury.

For some arthritis patients, lifting weights causes pain if the weight is moved through the entire range of motion. Rather than trying to work through the pain, try lifting the weight through a limited range of motion. You will still experience significant benefit from the lift, and gradually be able to push it further.

Strength-training do's and don'ts

▶ Warm up your muscles with a 5-10 minute aerobic workout on a stair stepper or treadmill, or take a walk. Your muscles will be better able to lift the load you will be asking them to handle after being warmed up.

▶ Focus on good form rather than on lifting heavy weights. Don't jerk weights into position with each lift and let them crash back down. Instead, lift and release slowly.

▶ Tighten the muscle you are working on throughout the entire range of motion of a particular exercise, maintaining the tension. This approach involves more muscle fibres in doing the work.

▶ Try to cover all major muscle groups during each workout.

▶ Vary your routine. There are more than 200 different types of strength-training exercise. After a couple of weeks, begin substituting new exercises for old ones.

▶ If you feel pain or odd feelings in your joints while exercising, stop. You may be doing the exercise wrongly or using too much weight.

▶ Gently stretch muscles after a workout.

Aerobic exercise

Exercises that increase your heart rate are called aerobic. More specifically, aerobic exercise is any activity that uses your large muscles in a repetitive fashion long enough to get your heart beating at 60 to 80 per cent of its maximum rate for at least 20, but preferably 30, minutes.

Aerobic exercise – which includes cycling, walking, swimming, skipping, rowing, roller-skating, ice-skating or even cross-country skiing, if you are able to find the snow – increases your overall fitness by training your heart and lungs to deliver oxygen more efficiently to the working muscles of the body. Since people with arthritis tend to be less active and therefore less fit, they usually have a lot to gain from aerobic exercise. Additionally, aerobic exercises that also involve weight bearing, such as walking or jogging, can help to lubricate and nourish the crucially important joint cartilage.

> **FACT** During the first six months of an exercise programme, it is best to lengthen your workouts gradually. Increase your sessions by no more than 5 minutes a month.

Some aerobic exercises do double-duty for arthritis patients, stretching and strengthening the joints. Swimming, for example, is both a good aerobic exercise and ideal for stretching. Walking and dancing are aerobic and also help to build strength in both the leg and thigh muscles.

To improve your aerobic capacity, try to exercise at between 60 and 80 per cent of the maximum heart rate for your age. This ideal range for aerobic exercising is known as your target heart rate. (See *Calculating your heart rate*, page 244.)

The aerobic exercises generally recommended for arthritis patients offer a good workout without putting a lot of pressure on your joints. They include walking, cycling, swimming, aerobic dancing, and aerobic pool exercises – all of which have been shown to produce definite benefits.

In one study, patients with painful hip or knee OA were randomly assigned to three treatment programmes – aerobic walking, aerobic pool exercises, or non-aerobic stretching exercises – for 12 weeks. Both of the aerobic groups showed significant gains in aerobic capacity compared with the stretching group, while all three groups showed similar lessening of joint pain and tenderness. And in case you fear that exercise will send you to the medicine cabinet for pain relief: none of the three groups increased its use of pain medication throughout the study period.

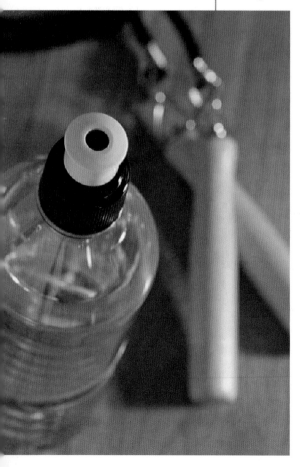

Exercise dropout?
How to keep in motion

Many people are eager to begin working out but more than half give up within three months. All too often, 'exercise dropouts' injure themselves by plunging in too aggressively rather than taking things slowly. But by taking basic precautions, you can minimize the risk that an exercise injury will derail your efforts to strengthen your joints.

Get a checkup If you are over 50, or haven't been physically active for many years, you should see your doctor to find out if your heart is up to the rigours of moderate exercise. A doctor's visit is also advisable if you know you have heart disease or one or more risk factors for heart disease, such as hypertension, diabetes or a high cholesterol level.

Even if vigorous exercise is out, you should work with your doctor in choosing stretching or other less-strenuous activity that can still be quite helpful.

Choose your exercises wisely Whether you design your own exercise programme or consult a physiotherapist or other expert, be sure to match your joints to the exercises that are most appropriate for them. If you have an arthritic shoulder, for example, include shoulder-stretching exercises but avoid strenuous weight lifting. If your knees are painful, then sprints are probably not in your future. By showing common sense in the exercises you choose, you can ensure that your programme will improve your arthritis without causing injuries.

Warm up As muscles warm up, they become more supple – easier to stretch and less likely to tear. So warming up prior to a workout can be quite important for avoiding injuries. A good warm-up usually takes 7-10 minutes – and even longer if, in the past, you've injured yourself while exercising. The idea is to raise your body temperature, elevate your heart rate and loosen up the muscles and joints so that they can withstand the stresses they'll soon be confronting.

continued on page 244

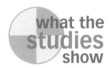

what the
studies
show

▷ A study has found that the great majority of older people don't need a stress test, in which heart function is measured as a patient works out on a treadmill. US researchers at Yale University concluded that the risk of heart attack from strenuous exercise has been overstated – and is outweighed by the health benefits that exercise can yield.

▷ For people with RA and other forms of inflammatory arthritis, aerobic exercise seems to offer a special bonus – reducing joint inflammation. Studies have shown that RA patients who completed aerobic exercise programmes had fewer inflamed joints than non-participants.

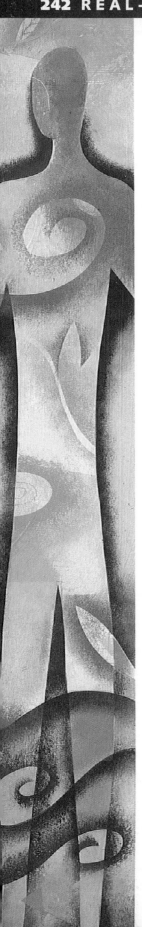

One active approach to arthritis

For Robina Lloyd of New Malden, Surrey, joining an exercise group for her arthritis was not a practical option. With a full-time job to hold down, a long commute, and a family to care for, it was simply too hard to fit a regular class into her busy schedule. Instead, with the help of her physiotherapist, she devised a personal regime to suit her life and available time.

Robina, 58, developed osteoarthritis in her arm quite early on in life, in her twenties, although she was not aware of what it was.

'At the age of fourteen I had a bad fall while ice skating. The cartilage in my knee was torn, and I had to have an operation to remove it – something that is rarely done these days.'

The operation was not a great success and Robina had continuing problems with her knee. Her neck then became a problem and she developed lower-back pain.

'But I kept on going because I was young enough to do so, and after all, I had two young children and a part-time job to cope with, as well as a house to restore!' Robina recalls.

Then things got worse. Robina's knee started letting her down, the backache became severe, and her feet were really very painful.

An arthroscopy operation helped Robina's knee for a while, but a visit to the chiropractor was a setback. This form of manipulations is far too violent for damaged joints.

A back-pain specialist recommended acupuncture, which worked well, but the pain relief lasted only for a short period of time.

A visit to her GP resulted in a series of sessions with a physiotherapist who recommended certain exercises for the back pain. Through trial and error, Robina has finally found the exercises that are right for her.

'I tried some aerobic exercises and soon discovered that they were not entirely suitable, as by then I had arthritis in both my knees, I was left in much more pain after the exercises, and simply couldn't get up or down.'

On the advice of her physiotherapist, Robina now does exercises before she gets out of bed.

'I lie flat on my back, knees bent, and swing my hips gently from side to side. Then I arch my back gently up and down.'

To help with the arthritis in her hands, Robina stretches them up above her head and then brings them back down with a circular movement. Then she turns her neck slowly from side to side.

'This means I can at least reach out for that first, reviving cup of tea. My bedside tea-maker is a godsend – it's perfect for people with stiff fingers, first thing in the morning.'

It's not always easy to exercise during the working day, of course, but again, Robina has found a way to deal with this.

'I can't do any formal exercises during the day,' Robina explains 'but I do stretch my back against a door in the office, and I insist on a half-hourly break during meetings. I also pull up my knee muscles, while I am sitting.'

Another tip that comes with Robina's recommendation is to imagine a balloon on a length of string, coming up out of the top of your head. It is lifting you and straightening your spine. This can help to keep your back straight.

'I also have one of those squidgy balls which I keep kneading with my hands during the day, in the office, as well as an ice pack in the fridge, to wrap around my hands when they get hot and painful.'

Robina's experience shows the importance of carefully and patiently working out what is right for you as an individual. Of course, each sufferer copes with arthritis in a different way. The right form of exercise and sensible management of your own time and strength can really help. 'I still work full time' says Robina. 'I hadn't expected to, but with a special ball-and-socket 'mouse' for my computer, and a cushion for my elbows, it has become quite possible for me to carry on almost as normal'.

Robina's advice to other arthritis sufferers is 'Don't struggle. Look for ways to do things that suit your particular requirements, and take advice on how life can be improved. I now enjoy watching ice skating on TV, even though I can no longer take an active part, and I am even learning to play the piano.'

Robina is not going to let arthritis stop her enjoying her life to the full, and being a wife, mother and grandmother.

'I start exercising before I even get out of bed,' says Robina.

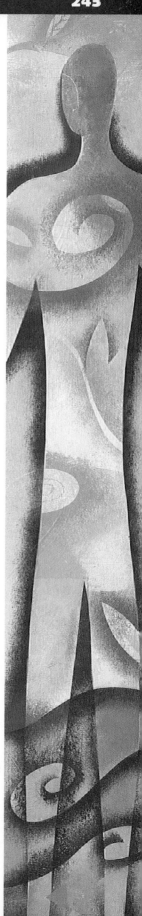

Calculating your heart rate

To calculate your maximum heart rate, do the following:

1 Subtract your age from 220. For example, if you're 55 years old, your maximum heart rate would be:
220 – 55 = 165 beats a minute.

2 Calculate the lower end of your target heart rate by taking 60 per cent of 165, which is 99.

3 Calculate the upper limit of your target heart rate by taking 80 per cent of 165, which is 132.

By this calculation, at age 55, your target heart range while exercising should be between 99 and 132 beats a minute. To improve your aerobic capacity, you should try to work out within your target heart range for 20-30 minutes three times a week.

You can monitor your heart rate by finding your pulse. Place your fingertips on the palm side of your wrist or lay them lightly against the side of your larynx (voice box). Count the pulses for 15 seconds, then multiply this number by four to get your pulse rate in beats a minute.

caution

Rest is certainly advisable if you have overdone things or if you're having a flare-up of joint pain (although even then you should probably do some gentle stretching exercises). But avoid the temptation to rest your joints for long periods of time, since the inactivity may actually increase pain and stiffness. Remember that not exercising poses far more risk to arthritic joints than doing proper exercises.

Good ways to warm up muscles include pedalling on a stationary bike, moderately fast walking or a spell of jogging on the spot.

Stretch Stretching is a useful prelude to exercise and also a vital form of exercise in its own right for people with arthritis. Contrary to standard wisdom, researchers have found that stretching before a workout does not decrease the risk of injury, but does help to reduce the pain and discomfort that can occur when stiff joints are made to move. People with arthritis should do stretching exercises each day or at least every other day. When stretching precedes other exercise, a 15-30 second stretch should suffice.

Ease into it For the first two weeks, maintain an easy, relaxed pace. Exercise for no more than 10 or 20 minutes at a time and no more than three or four times a week. You should expect a little muscle soreness when you embark on any exercise programme.

Soften the impact Arthritis patients should be especially careful to protect sensitive joints from unaccustomed jolts. So limit yourself to low-impact exercises such as walking, cycling or swimming, and try to work out on soft, smooth surfaces such as grass, or cushioned surfaces in a gym. In addition, proper footwear can be a big help in defusing the shocks of repeated impacts. Buy high-quality running or walking shoes from a good shoe shop that employs knowledgeable salespeople. You want shoes that are suited to your particular feet, so ask whether your feet underpronate (usually meaning you have high arches and need good arch support) or overpronate (meaning you probably have flat-feet and need a well-cushioned sole). Replace your shoes as soon as they seem to have lost some cushioning ability – even if the tread still looks new.

To further muffle the pounding, consider buying cushioned insoles for your shoes. One study found that wearing such insoles while walking can decrease the shock measured at the knee by nearly 50 per cent.

Listen to your senses You can expect some muscle soreness when you first start an exercise programme. But don't continue exercising if joint pain worsens, and be alert to these warning signs that you've overdone it:

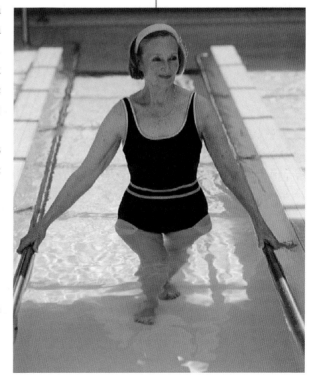

❍ Muscle or joint pain that lasts more than 2 hours after you've stopped exercising

❍ Unusually severe fatigue

❍ Increased muscle weakness

❍ Decreased range of motion of one or more joints

❍ Increased joint swelling

Splint it

When something – too much exercise, say – suddenly intensifies your joint pain, there is a tried and tested way to lower it: rest. And one of the oldest, most effective ways of doing that is with a splint.

Today's splints are lighter and sleeker than those of the past and made of plastic or a combination of plastic and rubber. They can be purchased over-the-counter or fitted, usually by an occupational therapist. One of the simplest splints is a slip-on type used to immobilize the joints of the fingers. (A variation is the silver-ring splint, which allows limited movement of the finger joints.) Splints can also be fitted to many other joints, such as the wrist or elbow.

Splints are never worn permanently; they are designed to be put on and taken off easily, as needed, and should be used for short-term relief only, as immobility is the enemy of arthritis sufferers. Sometimes a splint is worn during the day but your doctor may recommend wearing it only at night.

Water power You need water to replace fluids you lose through perspiration, while exercising, and to reduce the risk of muscle cramps. Try to drink two glasses of water 2 hours before you exercise, an additional glass every 20 minutes while you are exercising, and another glass or two within the hour after you stop exercising.

Cool down Suddenly stopping exercise can sharply reduce blood pressure, causing fainting or even a heart attack. So, just as it is essential to take time to warm up when you start, end each session with a cooling down period during which you spend a few minutes doing stretches and slow walking or some gentle callisthenics.

○ **FACT** Try to exercise when joints are least likely to feel stiff or fatigued, perhaps in the late morning or early afternoon. Early mornings or late evenings are not ideal.

Top 20 exercises to strengthen and stretch your muscles

Some exercises can increase flexibility as well as strengthen the muscles and other tissues that bend the joint. Most of the exercises described below fall into this two-for-one category.

These exercises can be done daily. Start gradually, doing two or three repetitions of each exercise; then slowly increase your number of repetitions until, for each exercise, you can do three sets of ten repetitions (30 repetitions in all) in one session.

Good moves for the knees

Quadriceps tighteners

- Lie on your back with your legs comfortably bent at the knee, then prop yourself up on your elbows and forearms.

- Extend one leg until it is straight, and then tighten the thigh muscle of your extended leg; note that this action should push the back of your knee down towards the floor. Then switch legs and repeat, to complete one repetition.

Foot lifts

- Place a firm pillow under one knee and lie flat on your back. (Bend your other leg comfortably at the knee, keeping the foot on the floor.)

- Without moving your knee off the pillow, slowly raise your foot until your leg is straight and then gently lower your foot to the floor. Switch legs and repeat.

Extend and flex

- Sit up straight in a chair with both feet flat on the floor.

- Slowly straighten one leg so that it is parallel with the floor, holding that position for 3 to 5 seconds.

- Bend your knee and slowly return your foot to the floor. Repeat with the other leg.

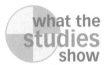

what the studies show

- In a US study, women who ate a moderately low-calorie diet and did either strength training or aerobic exercise lost more weight than women who just dieted. But those women who split their workout time between aerobic exercise and strength training lost the most weight of all.

Better biomechanics

Although exercise can help your joints and arthritis, poor posture and poor biomechanics can cancel out that good medicine. Here are some suggestions that can take the strain out of daily tasks:

- If you have arthritis of the hands, use an electric can opener rather than a manual model, and don't hold objects in a tight grip for extended periods. When holding anything, flex your fingers frequently.

- If reaching up hurts your shoulder, place frequently used items on lower shelves.

- Maintain good posture. It places the least stress on your joints.

- Use the largest joint possible to accomplish any task. Carry a shoulderbag rather than a clutch bag, because your shoulder joint is larger than your finger joints.

- Try to keep your joints extended rather than bent.

- Try not to stay in one position for a long period of time.

- If you have rheumatoid arthritis, avoid bending; arrange your rooms so that you reach up for items and use extended shoehorns that are easier on inflamed joints.

Reach for the stars

- Lie on your back with one leg comfortably bent at the knee and the other extended as straight as possible on the floor.

- Bend the knee of the straight leg, bringing it as far toward your chest as you can.

- Straighten that leg, making sure to push out with your heel, so that your foot points directly upward.

- Bend the knee back toward your chest and lower the leg to the floor.

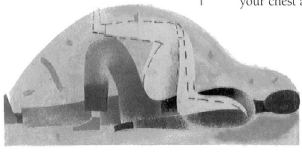

● Repeat again with the same leg, but this time push your leg out at a different angle. Repeat three to five times, extending your leg at a different angle each time. Then do the same routine with the other leg.

Quad builder

● Lie on your back with one leg bent and the other flat on the floor.

● Flex the foot of the flat leg (i.e., point your toes back toward your head), tighten your knee so the leg is straight, then lift that leg until your foot is 2ft off the floor.

● Count slowly to five, then lower the leg slowly, touching the floor with your calf first. Repeat with your other leg.

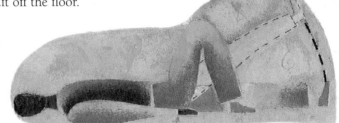

Medicine for the hips

Side leg lifts

● With your head resting on your arm, lie on your side with the leg you want to exercise on top. (Bend your bottom leg slightly to maintain balance.)

● Being careful to keep your top leg straight and without moving it forward, lift it about 2ft off the floor and then slowly lower it. Repeat with the other leg.

Hip rolls

● Lie on your back and extend both legs.

● Rotate one leg inward, then rotate it outward. Repeat with the other leg.

Thigh lifts

● Sit in a chair with both of your feet flat on the floor.

● Raise the knee of your affected leg as high as possible, then slowly lower it.

Arthritis profile

Theodore Roosevelt, Jr.

His father led the famous charge up San Juan Hill during the Spanish-American War and later became president. Theodore Roosevelt, Jr. also knew how to take charge; despite suffering from severe osteoarthritis of the hip, Brigadier General Roosevelt led his troops ashore during the Normandy Invasion – the only general to land with the first assault wave.

On D-Day, June 6, 1944, Roosevelt and his forces landed on Utah Beach. The landing crafts arrived nearly a mile south of their intended target, prompting Roosevelt to tell his men, 'We're going to start the war from right here'.

For the rest of D-Day – armed with only a pistol, walking with a cane due to his arthritis and while under constant enemy fire – Roosevelt repeatedly led groups of his men over a sea wall to positions inland.

General Omar N. Bradley, commander of the overall amphibious operation, would later describe this as the single bravest action he had ever seen.

In a letter to his wife on the eve of the invasion, Roosevelt had written: 'I go in with the assault wave and hit the beach at H-Hour. I'm doing it because it's the way I can contribute most. It steadies the young men to see me plodding along with my cane.'

For his 'valour and courage', Roosevelt was awarded the Congressional Medal of Honour, the highest military award possible in the armed forces of the United States of America.

Help for the neck

Stare down

▶ Looking straight ahead with your chin slightly dropped, bend your head forward, keeping your chin tucked in.

▶ Raise your head but don't bend your neck backwards.

Look both ways

▶ Begin by looking straight ahead, with your chin dropped slightly.

▶ Turn your head and look over your left shoulder.

▶ Then turn it so you're looking over your right shoulder.

Tick-tock

▶ Look straight ahead with your chin slightly dropped.

▶ As you continue staring straight ahead, bend your head sideways so that your ear moves toward your shoulder. (Don't lift your shoulder toward your ear.)

▶ Bend your head to the other side.

Stronger shoulders and elbows

Shoulder touch

▶ Sit or stand with your arms at your sides, palms facing backwards.

▶ Lift both arms forward to shoulder level with both palms facing down.

▶ Turn your palms up, and touch your fingertips to your shoulders, allowing your elbows to drop.

▶ Straighten arms at shoulder level, turning palms down.

▶ Lower your arms slowly, first to your side and behind your back, and then touch your palms together.

Shoulder circle

▶ Make sure both of your shoulders are relaxed as you look straight ahead.

▶ Roll both shoulders in circular movements – forward, up, backwards and down.

did you know

▶ Pain and stiffness in one joint often leads to problems in another. The ankle, for example, is rarely affected by osteoarthritis, but people with OA of the knee often develop ankles that are weak and have limited motion. The pain in their knee has caused them to walk more gingerly, and with less weight placed on the foot, the calf muscle grows weak and the ankle becomes stiff. For similar reasons, OA of the knee quite often leads to impaired hip motion as well, and vice versa.

Touch down

- ◗ Sit on a stool or other hard surface with your back straight, your feet flat on the floor, and your hands on your knees.

- ◗ Touch your stomach with your hands, keeping your elbows out to the side.

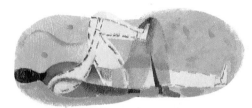

  - ◗ With elbows extended out to the sides, touch your shoulders, then touch behind your head.

  - ◗ Stretch both arms upward with your palms facing each other, then lower your arms back to your knees.

A supple back

Pelvic tilt

- ◗ Lie on your back, knees bent and feet flat on the floor.

- ◗ Press your back against the floor as you tighten your stomach. Hold this position for a count of ten, then relax.

Body curl

- ◗ As you flatten your back against the floor in the pelvic tilt position above, slowly bring your knees toward your chest, using your hands to pull your knees even closer. Hold this position for a count of ten, with your knees slightly apart as you do so.

- ◗ Slowly allow your feet to return to the floor.

Leg slides

- ◗ Starting in the pelvic-tilt position, slowly slide one foot away from you until your leg is straightened.

- ◗ Slowly pull it back to the bent-knee position, keeping your back pressed to the floor the entire time. Repeat with the other foot.

Curl and slide

- ◗ Lie on your back with your knees bent.

Taking a load off

Although exercise is the best way to protect your joints, there are aids take the pressure off stiff joints.

Walking stick Anyone who walks with a limp should consider using one; it protects the joints by taking weight off them and is helpful during a flare-up. Using it properly can relieve pressure on the hip joint by up to 50 per cent.

Bath and kitchen tips Elevated toilet seats with handles and bath boards can take stress off joints. In the kitchen special knives with L-shaped handles, cutting boards that hold foods firmly in place, and electric can openers and jar openers can help arthritis sufferers.

◉ Bring one knee toward your chest and hold it with both hands.

◉ With your back pressed to the floor, slowly slide your other foot along the floor until that leg is straight.

◉ With your back still pressed against the floor, slowly slide that leg back until it returns to the bent-knee position. Then switch legs and repeat.

The Buddha

◉ Sitting with your legs crossed in front of you, hold your feet with your hands.

◉ Slowly lean forward, moving your face toward the floor.

Chair bend

◉ Sit up straight in a chair, with your feet flat and your hands on your hips.

◉ Look directly ahead, and bend your trunk to one side.

◉ Return to the sitting-up-straight position, bend over to the other side, and then return to sitting up straight.

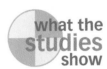

what the studies show

◉ Volunteers between 58 and 70 years old were asked to practice t'ai chi five days a week. After one year, volunteers experienced 15 to 20 per cent improvement in both aerobic capacity and knee strength.

Reduce the stress, to reduce the pain

Exercise is useful not just for its ability to help nurture cartilage and to help you to lose weight, but also for its well-known benefit of short-circuiting stress. Stress can be a big problem for arthritis patients, increasing their sensitivity to pain, tightening the muscles around their joints and hindering their movement.

Many studies have shown that regular exercise reduces anxiety, muscle tension and blood pressure – three key measures of stress – for at least several hours and possibly much longer, for healthy people as well as for those suffering from arthritis.

Two forms of exercise in particular – yoga and t'ai chi – may be especially useful for arthritis patients who are seeking to control and overcome anxiety and pain.

T'ai chi: ballet in slow motion

This ancient Chinese discipline could actually serve as a complete fitness programme, since its graceful, fluid movements manage to combine the three forms of exercise that lend a helping hand to arthritis patients: strength training, stretching and aerobic exercise. Several studies have shown that t'ai chi helps people to improve or maintain strength, joint flexibility, and balance, and can also boost aerobic capacity. But in addition, t'ai chi promotes a sense of well-being and relaxation that arthritis patients find especially helpful.

Tai chi consists of a series of movements, known as 'forms,' that resemble ballet in slow motion. As you perform these movements, you concentrate intently on both the movement and your breathing. The combination of these movements provides a workout for all the limbs and muscles. And since t'ai chi is gentle and low impact, it is ideally suited for people with arthritis – both osteoarthritis and rheumatoid arthritis.

Most teachers of t'ai chi believe that it takes a lifetime to truly master the discipline. If you don't have that long – and who does? – take several classes with an experienced instructor.

Alternatively, t'ai chi classes may be offered by your local health clubs, martial arts schools and community centre. Search the internet or look in the Yellow Pages for a t'ai chi instructor near you. You can also buy or rent videos that instruct you in t'ai chi.

> ◐ **FACT** T'ai chi doesn't seem to trigger rheumatoid arthritis symptoms. Researchers taught 20 people with RA a t'ai chi routine and supervised two hour-long sessions a week for ten weeks. None of them experienced any aggravation of symptoms.

Yoga – or how to stretch yourself healthy

The word yoga means 'union' and the practice of this Hindu discipline is aimed at uniting the body and mind with the soul. But whether or not you embrace the mystical aspects of yoga, you may find that it helps to relieve arthritis symptoms and offers valuable peace of mind. The basic elements of yoga are controlled breathing and various postures or positions such as the lotus position. Yoga helps arthritis patients because it involves stretching, extending and relaxing the limbs of the body.

Some yoga positions are virtually identical to the stretching exercises that physiotherapists recommend for arthritis patients. Others help to strengthen the muscles, tendons and ligaments that surround the joint. And almost all of them help to reduce stress and create a feeling of relaxation.

For best results with yoga, you should practise it regularly, for 45 minutes or an hour a day if possible. If you cannot spare that much time, shorter daily sessions lasting 15 minutes or so are preferable to longer sessions that you do just once or twice a week. Set aside a time and space for your yoga exercises, and endeavour to relax and put the clamour of the world out of your mind as you perform them.

The best way to learn yoga is in a class with a qualified, experienced instructor. Your local community centre probably offers an introductory course, and videos are also available. You will also find yoga classes advertised in your local newspaper, on the internet and in the Yellow Pages.

> **caution**
>
> Beware of yoga instructors who make extravagant claims about the potential health benefits of yoga. The best courses are those that begin with the simplest and safest positions and then become gradually more rigorous.

The final word

If you've followed most of the advice in this book, you may be wondering when you will start to feel better. Perhaps you already do, but there may be some unlucky people who feel disappointed that all the talk of self-empowerment has not yet made a difference in their life.

Be patient Our advice is just wait a little longer. As you follow the take-charge plan, remember that you alone can provide the most important ingredient for success: patience. You may well be in pain and your joints probably feel stiff and creaky. Above all, you want to feel better. You can, but it may take time.

In all likelihood, your arthritis developed over the course of many years. Just as it takes time to break a bad habit, it may take a while – perhaps several months of effort on your part – before you sense that your take-charge efforts have started to turn things round and that you have gained control of your condition.

In addition to patience, the other ingredient that you need is perseverance. No arthritis treatment will help absolutely everyone, but most people should be able to find a particular therapy, or combination of therapies, that will prove helpful. You may not find it immediately, but you owe it to yourself to keep trying.

Remember the example of Gill Boreham (on page 158). During the course of several years, she tried virtually all arthritis drugs to treat her arthritis. Through it all she remained patient and persevered, and she finally found a drug that was fairly new on the market and that has made all the difference for her.

Gill also did something else crucial to taking charge: she put a lot of effort into informing herself about her disease and her treatment options. Medical knowledge is never static – and, in the case of arthritis, major advances have occurred over the past few years. There is no reason to doubt that they will continue.

No time is a good time to develop arthritis, but with recent medical advances and the proven effectiveness of the take-charge approach, people with arthritis can now live more fulfilling, less painful lives than ever before.

We've come a long way in our efforts to successfully manage arthritis, and the best may yet be to come.

Resource guide

Organizations for patients and professionals

Arthritis and Musculoskeletal Alliance
41 Eagle Street
London WCIR 4TL
Tel. 020 7242 3313
www.boneandjointdecade.org
Umbrella group bringing together support groups, professional bodies and research organizations in the field of arthritis and musculoskeletal conditions. Raises awareness and promotes development of treatment.

Arthritis Care
18 Stephenson Way
London NWI 2HD
Tel. 020 7380 6500
www.arthritiscare.org.uk
Offers social and welfare assistance with arthritis and runs the 'Challenging Arthritis' courses.

Arthritis Research Campaign
PO Box 177
Chesterfield S41 7TQ
Tel. 0870 850 5000
www.arc.org.uk
Funds medical research into arthritis and produces free literature on arthritis.

British Acupuncture Council (BAcC)
63 Jeddo Road
London W12 9HQ
Tel. 020 8735 0400
www.acupuncture.org.uk
BAcC publishes a list of qualified practitioners and provides general information on acupuncture.

British Association for Counselling and Psychotherapy
BACP House
35-37 Albert Street
Rugby CV21 2SG
Tel. 0870 443 5252
www.bacp.co.uk
Promoter, supervisor and regulator of counsellors and psychotherapists in the UK.

British Chiropractic Association
Blagrave House
17 Blagrave Street
Reading RG1 IQB
Tel. 0118 950 5950
www.chiropractic-uk.co.uk
The BCA represents 70 per cent of internationally accredited UK chiropractors. It aims to encourage and maintain high standards of conduct, practice, education and training within the profession in this country and has lists of accredited practitioners.

British Holistic Medical Association
59 Lansdown Place
Hove BN3 IFL
Tel. 01273 725951
www.bhma.org
Promotes principles and practice of holistic medicine. Publishes *Holistic Health* – a journal available to members.

British Nutrition Foundation
High Holborn House
52-54 High Holborn
London WC1V 6RQ
www.nutrition.org.uk
Promotes nutritional wellbeing in partnership with academic and research institutes, the food industry, educators and the government.

British Osteopathic Association
Langham House West
Luton LU1 2NA
Tel. 01582 488455
www.osteopathy.org
An organization representing professional osteopaths, which can also help you to find an osteopath in your area.

British Reflexology Association
Monks Orchard
Whitbourne WR6 5RB
Tel. 01886 821207
www.britreflex.co.uk
Publishes a general information sheet on reflexology. For a list of registered practitioners, send an SAE and £2.

British Society for Rheumatology
41 Eagle Street
London WC1R 4TL
Tel. 020 7242 3313
www.rheumatology.org.uk
Professional organization for people working in rheumatology and related fields in the UK. Its objective is to advance the science and practice of rheumatology and to promote study and research through scientific meetings and education courses.

Children's Chronic Arthritis Association (CCAA)
Amber Gate
City Walls Road
Worcester WR1 2AH
Tel. 01905 745595
www.ccaa.org.uk
Run by parents and professionals to provide help and information for children with arthritis, their families and professionals involved in their care.

Contact a Family
209-211 City Road
London EC1V 1JN
Tel. 020 7608 8700
Helpline: 0808 808 3555
(Monday to Friday 10am to 4pm)
www.cafamily.org.uk
The organization provides support and advice for families with disabled children and can often put families in touch with each other.

Disability Rights Commission
DRC Helpline
FREEPOST MID02164
Stratford upon Avon
CV37 9BR
Helpline 08457 622 633.
www.drc-gb.org
Independent body set up by the government to eliminate discrimination against disabled people and promote equality of opportunity. The commission can provide advice and information for disabled people, employers and service providers.

Family Fund Trust
PO Box 50
York YO1 9ZX
Tel. 0845 130 45 42
www.familyfund.org.uk
The Trust helps families of disabled and ill children by giving grants and providing information on benefits, holidays and transport and other issues related to the care of the child. Grants are available for a range of items including specialist equipment, holidays and driving lessons. Most of the Trust's publications can be downloaded from their web site.

Fibromyalgia Association
PO Box 206
Stourbridge DY9 8YL
Helpline: 0870 220 1232
(Monday to Friday 10am to 4pm)
www.ukfibromyalgia.com
Promotes awareness of FM and provides
information and advice to sufferers
and their families and medical information
for professionals, as well as a national helpline.

Food Standards Agency
Aviation House
125 Kingsway
London WC2B 6NH
Tel. 020 7276 8000
www.foodstandards.gov.uk
Independent food safety watchdog set
up by the government to protect the
public's health and consumer interests
in relation to food.

**General Council for Massage
Therapy**
46 Millmead Way
Hertford SG14 3YH
Tel. 01992 537637
www.gcmt-uk.org
The lead body to promote, regulate and
research massage therapy in the UK.

Hughes Syndrome Foundation
The Rayne Institute
St Thomas' Hospital
London SE1 7EH
Tel. 020 7960 5561
www.hughes-syndrome.org
The foundation provides information
on Hughes Syndrome (Antiphospholipid
Syndrome or 'sticky blood') and the
work of the Foundation.

Institute for Complementary Medicine
PO Box 194
London SE16 7QZ
Tel. 020 7237 5165
www.icmedicine.co.uk
Encourages awareness and provides
information about complementary medicines.
Publishes a register of complementary
practitioners. For details, send an SAE.

Lady Hoare Trust
1st Floor
89 Albert Embankment
London SE1 7TP
Tel. 020 7820 9989
www.ladyhoaretrust.org.uk
The Trust gives practical help to children
suffering from Juvenile Idiopathic Arthritis
(JIA) and severe limb disabilities and their
families via a network of specially trained
fieldworkers as well as financial help in
the form of small grants.

Lupus UK
St James House,
Eastern Road,
Romford RM1 3NH
Tel. 01708 731251
www.lupusuk.com
Offers support, advice and counselling and
promotes awareness of the disorder.

National Ankylosing Spondylitis Society
PO Box 179
Mayfield
East Sussex TN20 62L
Tel. 01435 873527
www.nass.co.uk
Founded by patients, physiotherapists and
doctors 20 years ago, it informs and educates
to provide for efficient management of AS.

National Association for Colitis and Crohn's Disease
4 Beaumont House
Sutton Road
St Albans AL1 5HH
Information line: 0845 1302233
www.nacc.org.uk
Provides advice, support and information about association's activities nationwide.

National Institute of Medical Herbalists
56 Longbrook Street
Exeter EX4 6AH
Tel. 01392 426022
www.nimh.org.uk
Provides general information on herbal medicine along with a full list of qualified herbal practitioners.
Send an SAE for details.

Pain Concern
PO Box 13256
Haddington EH41 4YD
Listening-ear Helpline: 01620 822572
(Monday to Friday 9am to 5pm, and Friday evening 6.30pm to 7.30pm)
www.painconcern.org.uk
Provides information and support for pain sufferers and those who care for them.

Pain Society
21 Portland Place
London W1B 1PY
Tel. 020 7631 8870
www.painsociety.org
Representative body for all UK professionals involved in the management and understanding of pain. Offers general information on chronic pain and details of UK pain clinics.

St Thomas' Lupus Trust
The Rayne Institute
St Thomas' Hospital
London SE1 7EH
Tel. 020 7922 8197
www.lupus.org.uk
The charity which funds lupus research at St Thomas', results of which have made a major contribution to the increased survival of lupus patients.

Society of Teachers of the Alexander Technique
1st Floor, Linton House
39-51 Highgate Road
London NW5 1RS
0845 230 7828
www.stat.org.uk
The society's aim is to ensure high standards of teacher training and professional practice. Provides a full list of teachers.

UK Tai Chi Association
PO Box 159,
Bromley BR1 3XX
Tel. 020 8289 5166
www.taichi-europe.com

Web sites

British National Formulary (BNF)
www.bnf.org
Authoritative and practical information on the selection and clinical use of medicines.

NHS Direct
www.nhsdirect.nhs.uk
Health information supplied by the National Health Service.

Index

Credits

Photography
4-5 Photodisc   10 Photodisc
14 Spinning Egg Design
17 Photo Alto   28 Photodisc
35 Photo Alto   41 Stock
Market   42 Photodisc
52 Stock Market
66 Photodisc   81 Photo
Alto   84 Photodisc
90 Photodisc
101 Comstock
105 Imagesource
112 Corbis   113 Alamy
Images/ Imagesource
114 Photodisc   120 Eyewire
134 Photodisc
149 Comstock   154 Eyewire
160 Eyewire   170 Photodisc
174 Corbis   191 Photodisc
198 Corbis   201 Photodisc
208 Photodisc
210 Photodisc
214 Dynamic Graphics
218 Digital Stock
221 Eyewire   223 Photodisc
226 Photodisc   232 Stock
Market   240 Photodisc
245 Eyewire   254 Photodisc

Illustration
7, 12, 13, 18, 21, 30, 58, 61,
71, 74, 92, 97, 116, 124,
126, 136, 158, 165, 174,
179, 187, 201, 206, 216,
226, 230, 242, 248, 249,
252 Linda Frichtell
33 Hugo Cruz
39, 47 Articulate Graphics

Taking Charge of Arthritis was published by
The Reader's Digest Association Limited, London
First edition copyright © 2004

The Reader's Digest Association Limited,
11 Westferry Circus, Canary Wharf, London E14 4HE

Adapted from *Taking Charge of Arthritis* © 2001
originated by the editorial team of The Reader's Digest
Association Inc., USA

We are committed to both the quality of our
products and the service we provide to our customers.
We value your comments, so please feel free to contact
us on **08705 113366** or via our web site at:
www.readersdigest.co.uk
If you have any comments or suggestions
about the content of our books, email us at:
gbeditorial@readersdigest.co.uk

Paperback edition
Copyright © 2004 Reader's Digest Association
Far East Limited
Philippines Copyright © 2004 Reader's Digest Association
Far East Limited

Concept Code: US 4011/H-US
Book Code: 400-186-01
ISBN: 0 276 42849 8
Oracle Code: 250001599S.00.24